.....I KNOW KA-RAZY....
REJECTING THE
CAPITALIST ROAD TO
TWISTED MENTAL HEALTH

BERNARD NICOLAS

.....I KNOW KA-RAZY....
REJECTING THE CAPITALIST ROAD TO TWISTED MENTAL HEALTH

© **2026 Bernard Nicolas, LMFT**

All rights reserved. No part of this manuscript may be reproduced, stored in a retrieval system, or transmitted in any form or by any means—electronic, mechanical, photocopying, recording, or otherwise—without the prior written permission of the author and/or publisher, except in the case of brief quotations used in articles or reviews.

DISCLAIMER: This book is intended for informational and educational purposes only. It is not intended to provide medical, psychological, legal, or other professional advice. The content reflects the author's personal views and experiences and should not be interpreted as a substitute for professional consultation, diagnosis, or treatment. Always seek the advice of a qualified professional with any questions you may have regarding a medical or mental health condition. The author and publisher disclaim any liability arising directly or indirectly from the use or application of the information contained in this book.

ISBN - Print: 979-8-9941680-0-4
e-book: 979-8-9941680-1-1

CONTENTS

– Introduction
1

1 – 20/20 - It's Normal to Have Issues
7

2 – Mangled Care
21

3 – Coping Strategies
43

4 – Concepts of Mental Health
61

5 – Mental Health as Public Health
75

6 – Guidelines for Good Mental Health
87

7 – The Capitalist Road: Artificial Sugar
99

8 — Dare to Dream
109

9 — Psychology of Liberation
121

10 — Maintainting Mental Health
133

— About the Author
145

— Acknowledgments
146

— Photo Credits
147

— End Notes
149

"He who has health has hope,
and he who has hope has everything."[1]
African Proverb (Anonymous)

INTRODUCTION

We live in a time that many people would describe as "complete insanity." We have a population that is thoroughly polarized, a President who is a convicted criminal and seems to be severely mentally ill, and a plethora of extremist individuals whose desperation drives them to suicidal acts and/or vicious violence against others. A mainstream publication (*Newsweek*) recently published an article quoting various experts about the possibility of "civilizational collapse." The piece quotes historian Mike Duncan as he describes the U.S. as an empire that is past its peak:

> Everybody has a shelf-life. Eventually you do get into some sort of decline phase...is this thing pushing itself toward some sort of terminal failure? Yeah, sure feels like it...When systems can no longer adapt to their present circumstances, that's the kind of incompetence that leads to total and complete social upheaval.[2]

Part of the purpose of this book is to affirm that it is appropriate to begin to think about alternatives to the capitalist system we have been living with. Believing we cannot change the system, someone who pays attention to the present trends could easily become severely depressed about the future.

Partly because of my philosophical orientation and partly because it is the only way to maintain my mental health, I choose to see current times as a period of transition. We are actively moving from a stage of dying capitalism to one where the political economy will prioritize the wellbeing of the planet and its inhabitants. Perhaps someone will come up with a catchy new name for the new economic system. But whatever we end up calling it, it will be important not to pretend we are re-inventing the wheel. Many brilliant thinkers have been working on and writing about this potentially bright future. In this writing, I will be perfectly satisfied with socialism as defined by economist Richard Wolff,

> In socialism, the whole community of people served by, and living with, or in, an economy participate democratically in producing and distributing goods and services... Socialism accomplishes the transition from capitalism by rebuilding the economy from the bottom up.[3]

The famous line from a James Brown song ("The Big Payback") says, "I don't know karate, but I know ka-razy."[4] The implication is that "ka-razy" is equal to or more dangerous than karate. There is also an implication that, when necessary (such as when it's time for payback), "ka-razy" is just the right thing. This is a book about how we can reject the mangled care we have been receiving, embrace mental health, understand the difference between unhealthy and healthy coping strategies, and ultimately how we can strive to have a culture that is more nurturing than ka-razy.

Some of the ideas presented here are not new. German psychologist Erich Fromm, in his book *The Sane Society*, pointed out that good mental health is directly related to our connection to other human beings: "The necessity to unite with other living beings, to be related to them, is an imperative need on the fulfillment of which man's sanity depends."[5]

British scholar and psychotherapist James Davies, in his book *Sedated: How Modern Capitalism Created our Mental Health Crisis*, points out how over-reliance on psychotropic medication has failed, and how capitalism has depoliticized, pathologized, and commodified suffering.[6] Davies also believes that it will ultimately require a new economic paradigm to fundamentally change the current system. He also believes that consumers and providers of mental health services can unite to lead that change.

Ironically, the vast majority of books about mental health only address how individuals can work on their own mental health, as if we can be completely healthy in an environment that tries to detract from our mental health in myriad ways every day.

Human beings have a fundamental need for self-efficacy. Self-efficacy was defined by psychologist Albert Bandura as, "confidence in one's ability to influence events and outcomes in one's environment."[7] These days, many—if not most—of us do not feel that confidence. It's not about actual control of our environment. It's about believing that we can influence our environment enough to live a happy and healthy life. One of my clients was a middle-school history teacher for 25 years. He was proud to have taught many students who went on to become successful adults, and who were very grateful that his class had a profound impact on them. However, by the time the second Trump term came around, this devoted teacher found himself facing a school system that clearly had other priorities than teaching kids. This teacher's house was completely destroyed by rainwater because the city and county where he lived did not take the proper steps to effectively drain rainwater from the hill where he lived. The teacher sued the city and county but had no way of knowing if he could win or how long it would take to be reimbursed for the property that had been his biggest life investment. Of course, home insurance did not cover damage from flooding. So, the teacher decided to retire early and move out of state. He was saddened by the fact that he no longer knew how to explain to his middle school students how the political system was supposed to promote democracy and the balance of powers.

We live in a time of mental health crisis, at both the individual and public health levels. Since the pandemic of 2020, many more individuals have sought help through mental health counseling. At the same time, highly qualified professionals argue that the President of the United States suffers from one of the worse forms of mental illness, a personality disorder.[8] This same President helped to perpetrate a genocidal war, then wanted a Nobel Peace Prize for allegedly helping to end the genocide. Within the field of clinical psychology, personality disorders are considered among the most difficult issues to manage. That is because people with personality disorders, especially narcissists, often lack insight regarding their own issues.

Mass shootings in the U.S. from 2020 to 2024 averaged 600 per year, almost two per day.[9] Shocking news stories pop up routinely, such as a man in Pennsylvania who in 2025 shot his father (with whom he disagreed politically), decapitated him, and displayed the severed head in a video on social media.[10] There was also the astrology-influencer mom from California who in 2024 abandoned her two daughters on the side of the freeway, then killed herself by crashing her car into a tree—all because she believed that a solar eclipse was a sign of a "spiritual apocalypse."[11] Neither the California mom nor the Pennsylvania man had a history of mental health diagnosis or treatment.

Of course, some perpetrators of mass shootings have had prior contact with the mental health system. The Virginia Tech student who killed 33 people in 2007 is one such example. He was hospitalized a couple of years before the shooting on suspicion of being suicidal and was even court-ordered to undergo outpatient treatment—but it did not prevent him from killing 33 people.

It is pointless to seek ways of reducing mass shootings or suicides without first addressing the need to fundamentally change the system that created—and continues to foster—failing methods of mental health care promotion and delivery. This book is a common sense approach to explaining why and how we can commit to the necessary fundamental changes.

CHAPTER 1

20/20 - IT'S NORMAL TO HAVE ISSUES

BERNARD NICOLAS

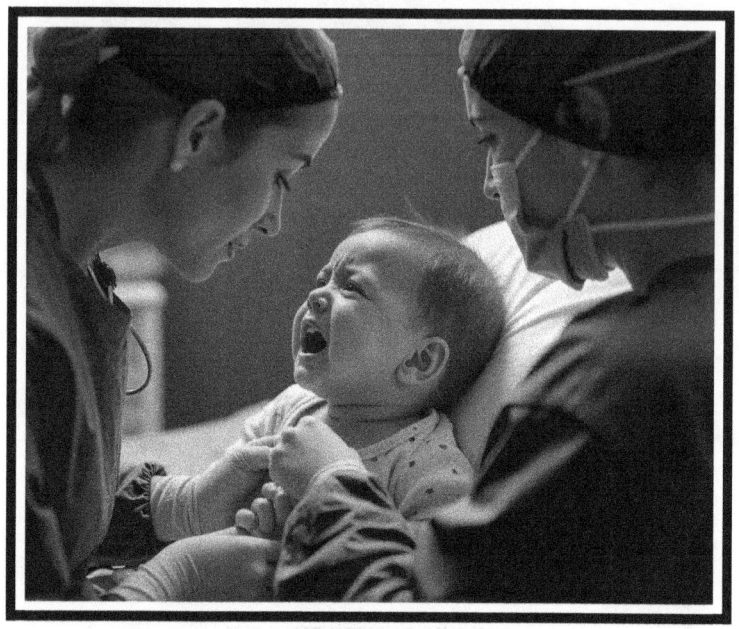

> **i** t's important to recognize that the vast majority of mental health issues are either caused or aggravated by "family."

Unlike a lot of people, I was blessed with a reasonably "normal" childhood. No major traumas, nor wretched economic conditions, nor parents with severe mental illnesses distorted my ability to reach into adulthood with promise and potential. In fact, my family adapted well to immigrating from the poorest to the richest economy in our hemisphere. My siblings and I did well in school, and we all received scholarships to attend University of California campuses.

Nevertheless, I developed mental health issues that caused me to qualify as "ka-razy" for 20 years. My primary issue turned out to be one called alcoholism. Like a lot of other chronic illnesses, alcoholism comes with a lot of denial. Even though my consumption of alcohol was affecting my relationships, my employability, and my self-esteem, I remained in denial about it for more than 10 years. The denial continued even after I reached a point where I had a loaded revolver in hand and I wanted to blow my brains out. I talked myself out of pulling the trigger because I could not think of a way to avoid my children seeing my corpse when they came home from school. Yet, even though I was under the influence of alcohol throughout this suicidal episode, it never occurred to me that alcoholism was the primary contributor to my depression. I thought it was because I could not find a job and that my attempt to move to Africa had failed.

But eventually, I was blessed to hit "bottom," seek treatment, and be able to turn my life around. Thank God there was well-developed treatment and support available so that I could learn how to manage my chronic illness very well.

After I was 12 years sober, I returned to graduate school and earned a Master's in Clinical Psychology. I did 3,000 hours of supervised practice, passed two rigorous exams to become a licensed mental health therapist, and helped other "crazies" heal for the next 20 years. These 40 years of experience have provided me with the "20/20" vision that encourages me to share what I have come to understand about mental health and what it might take to improve it substantially on both an individual and community level.

And yet, here I am writing a book in a time when far more people get their knowledge from watching YouTube than reading books. That is simply because I don't know how to present a complex issue such as mental health in a YouTube video. Perhaps once the book is published, my next challenge will be to turn it into a series of video presentations. I know that one of these presentations would offer my simple definition of good mental health:

> Good mental health is knowing what your issues are and what you need to do to manage them.

This definition clearly suggests that good mental health is not about the absence of issues. Quite the contrary, it is completely normal for human beings to have "issues." We start having them from the moment we are born. Then we discover new issues as we seek to define our identity and confront other challenging concerns.

.....I KNOW KA-RAZY.... REJECTING THE CAPITALIST ROAD TO TWISTED MENTAL HEALTH

Imagine yourself floating in warm liquid inside the womb. All your needs are met and ideally your mother is free of stress, has good prenatal care, and enjoys good nutrition. Suddenly, with no eviction notice, you are pushed out to a soundtrack of screams and pains, and forced to breathe air. Once you are over the shock of wondering what happened to your nice, peaceful environment, you see a bunch of large people and you begin to wonder which one of them is going to take care of you. Eventually one or two are identified as caregivers. But they keep on leaving the room (which to an infant is the equivalent of abandonment), and this stresses you out a lot. Sometimes, even though you scream as loudly as you can, no one comes to check on you. All of this adds up to what clinicians refer to as "attachment issues."

An entire theoretical framework in clinical psychology has been built around issues of attachment. The basic idea is that the kind of attachment we have in early childhood affects all of our future relationships. The theory posits that attachment can be secure, insecure, or something in-between. Most of us do not end up with a totally secure sense of attachment, if only because our parents have to work, and/or are stressed out by financial issues, lack of support, and perhaps their own mental health issues. It should be mentioned that many new parents are totally unprepared to deal with the demanding needs of a newborn who wants to eat every two hours or so.

Generally, we tend to romanticize family relations—but it's important to recognize that the vast majority of mental health issues are either caused or aggravated by "family." Since most parents are not able to provide a consistently healthy and peaceful environment for their children, it is understandable that most of us will have attachment or anxiety issues from an early age. When and if medical technology allows it, perhaps requiring some minimal preparation prior to parenting would be helpful—something at least equivalent to the preparation required to get a driver's license (having to study a pamphlet and pass both a written and practical test). Better yet, having a system that provides free access to mental health support to all, whether or not they choose to be parents, would be great. Such a system could offer regular mental health check-ups the same way we do physical health check-ups. When people decide to become parents, enter a career in policing, run for president, or open a gun store, it would be reasonable to have a more extensive evaluation—the same way we assess the mental and physical health of astronauts or airline pilots, for example.

Once we survive the attachment issues, then come the "identity issues." This particular set of issues involves gender, race, sexuality and class. To begin with, let's make a distinction between sex, gender, gender identity, and sexuality.

- "Sex" refers to biological characteristics such as male or female reproductive organs and combinations of chromosomes. Yet even these biological elements exist on a spectrum rather than being strictly binary. Some people have both male and female sexual organs at birth, or their chromosomes function differently from the typical biochemistry of someone with the sexual organ they have.
- "Gender" is a socially-constructed notion of how people with a particular set of biological elements should behave. For example, humans with a longer appendage called a penis instead of the shorter clitoris are not supposed to play with dolls and should avoid crying in public.
- "Gender identity" is a person's internal sense of self which may or may not correspond with the sex assigned at birth. And again, gender identity is clearly on a spectrum as there are vast differences within the group of people who identify as male; just as there are with those who identify as female.
- "Sexuality" has to do with the kind of people one is attracted to and the sexual behavior that results from such attraction. And once again there is a wide range of sexuality or sexual orientation.

Some people find all of these categories too complicated or confusing. Others prefer to think there are only two sexes, each with a proper identity and sexuality, and that any variations from that are simply freaks. The diversity that exists in humans is real. The challenge of social systems is to be able to accommodate and even embrace the diversity, so that everyone has a chance to feel included and treated with equal dignity. Those who want to oversimplify reality are likely not pursuing good mental health. Such oversimplified ideas can not only harm the person holding them, but those with whom that person interacts, especially if they have influence over children. Imagine a father who emotionally abuses his nominally male child because that child is not acting in a manner the father perceives as "man" enough. How many homophobic individuals have taken their insanity to the extreme and murdered gay, lesbian, or trans people? There can never be a well-thought-out reason to commit such a murder. Perpetrators of physical abuse or murder of others are driven by their own internal issues and not by the external issues they claim to be motivated by.

To me it makes sense that all humans have a strong need to be accepted. Top scholars of "belonging research" have indicated that "we called belonging a 'need' rather than merely a 'desire' because people who fail to satisfy it suffer various mental and physical health deficits."[12] Well-respected scholars, Baumeister and Leary, determined that, although much of human anxiety has to do with fear of death or injury, "by far the biggest theme was [fear of] being socially rejected, excluded, or otherwise condemned to being alone."[13] Just as with cops involved in dangerous operations or soldiers in battle, early humans felt that not being fully accepted could mean life or death. A soldier or fellow cop who does not like you, may not "have your back" the way he or she would for someone considered a full member of the "in-group." Some unhealthy people define their "in-group" in terms of hate toward others, or they blame others for the loss of status of their in-group. White supremacists are an example of this kind of thinking.

> One thing white supremacy terrorists likely have in common, other than being white, is that they are deeply afraid of loss—loss of the way life used to be, the way they want it to be once again. They see their future threatened by people of color and those who support them.[14]

Race has certainly been used as a difference ripe for exploitation. Scientifically speaking, a distinct race can only exist as an isolated gene pool. And with the amount of interaction that happens on our planet today, there are no completely isolated gene pools. Nevertheless, many systems and societies have used features identified as race characteristics to create arbitrary distinctions that can be used to deny certain groups their rights or to grant special rights to others. Cultural differences have also been exploited. And even within cultures, differences such as skin tone have been exploited to create differences in access to resources.

It is sad and pitiful that in recent years in the U.S., the slogan "Black Lives Matter" had to become popular. It reminds me of the famous picture from the Civil Rights Era of Black men wearing sandwich boards with big letters saying, "I am a man." If we did not live in a racist capitalist society, these slogans would seem trite and ridiculous. In his speech on May 29, 1964, to the Militant Labor Forum in New York City, Malcolm X said, "You can't have capitalism without racism." In fact, U.S. capitalism was built from the profits of the slave trade and the genocide against the native people who had thrived in so-called North America before the white man arrived. The reality of life under capitalism today is that the socio-political phenomenon of racism is very real. From a mental health point of view, parents of children of color in the U.S. must carefully support their children's self-esteem and sense of safety as they confront discrimination and learn about police killings of unarmed people of color.

In a 2019 policy statement, the American Academy of Pediatrics acknowledged that "the impact of racism has been linked to birth disparities and mental health problems in children and adolescents."[15] The same policy statement goes on to point out that racism causes chronic stress and that "prolonged exposure to stress hormones, such as cortisol, lead to inflammatory reactions that predispose individuals to chronic disease."[16] People who study racism realize that the primary issue is not so much the individual racist thoughts and attitudes that one or more persons may have, but the unequal allocation of power among groups defined by race and the lack of self-determination experienced by cultural groups whose identity is primarily defined by notions of race. If everyone truly had equal access to quality mental health support as well as equal access to top-notch education and employment, then racist attitudes could be discussed in a context that is about humanity and community, and not about one group having more power or privilege than another.

In light of the above then, identity issues, particularly under capitalism, are not only psychological issues but they have direct consequences in terms of access to resources and social power based on group affiliation.

The capitalist notion of "social media" seems to have created a great pressure among young people to determine their identities. Young men and women seem to have an urgency to decide if they are gay, straight, bisexual, Black, white, biracial, asexual, non-binary, or whatever. This pressure seems to exist even when there is no reason for it. For example, some teens who are not sexually active and probably will not be for five years or more seem to feel an immediate need to decide what their sexuality should be.

Interestingly, with all the attention paid to other categories of social distinction, "class identity" is not talked about as much in modern capitalist liberal culture. That is because the ruling class tends to benefit from propagating the myth that anyone can achieve any level of wealth they want if they are just willing to work hard for it. This myth has disastrous psychological consequences for people who come to believe that they must be inferior somehow if they are not able to achieve a certain level of wealth. The fact that class identity is not adequately discussed also prevents young people (who are otherwise very concerned about their identity) from finding out the social and economic impact of the choices they make. For example, having a large tattoo on your face or failing to acquire a college-level vocabulary is bound to influence what jobs you will be considered for.

Similarly, the socio-economic or "class conditions" you grow up in tend to determine the quantity or type of trauma you are likely to experience. Those same conditions also tend to determine your awareness of or access to good quality mental health. For example, in some Black or Brown communities, asking a random group of fifth graders if they know someone who has been shot to death will result in a majority of raised hands. Yet in those same communities where children are exposed to violent trauma (and therefore PTSD) there is little access to good quality mental health. One large study of Black people living in low-resource communities came to the conclusion that "while about 6 percent of the general population, and about 7 percent to 14 percent of veterans will be diagnosed with PTSD in their lifetimes, our research has shown that lifetime rates of PTSD in Black individuals living in urban low-resourced neighborhoods is 46 percent."[17] The point of this example is that it's not just being Black that can cause mental health issues in the U.S., but being impacted by race and class discrimination together can have an impact that is greater than the sum of the parts.

Overall, while it is normal to have issues, most people are made to think they should either not have issues, they should just "get over it," or they should "get some help"—as though help was readily and affordably available to all. We need to keep in mind that it is impossible for someone to seek help if they don't realize they need it. Promotion of mental health not only requires that we recognize and face our issues, but that we need to understand what mental health is. Most people know what some mental illness might look like or that certain behavior patterns are "kray-kray," but they don't have any real sense of what good mental health really means. That is most likely because instead of useful health care information, we have been recipients of "mangled care."

BERNARD NICOLAS

MANGLED CARE

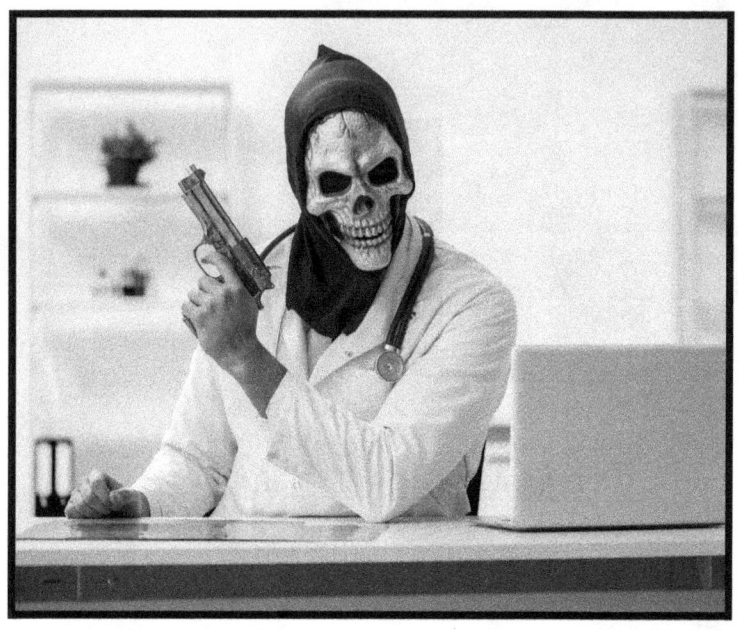

Ninety percent of U.S. adults say the U.S. is experiencing a mental health crisis.

There is plenty of evidence to illustrate the dire state of mental health on the planet in general and in the U.S. in particular:

- 90% of U.S. adults say the U.S. is experiencing a mental health crisis.[18]

- Every 40 seconds of every day someone somewhere in the world dies by suicide—it is the leading cause of death for people under 25.[19]
- In 2016, there were more than twice as many suicides as homicides in the U.S, a country with a high homicide rate compared to the rest of the world.[20]

These three bullet points alone already suggest how far we have to go to be a mentally healthy planet.

When we look at definitions of mental health, we realize that the challenge we face is far greater than simply radically reducing the suicide rate. According to a report from the Surgeon General of the U.S.,

> Mental Health is [also] defined as the successful performance of mental function, resulting in productive activities, fulfilling relationships with other people, and the ability to adapt to change and to cope with adversity; from early childhood until late life. Mental health is the springboard of thinking and communication skills, learning, emotional growth, resilience, and self-esteem.[21]

In the history of mental health treatment in Eurocentric cultures, only recently has the focus tried to shift from "mental illness" to "mental health." The difference between the two approaches is mostly similar to the shift in perceptions of physical health. We now largely accept the importance of preventive measures, such as regular check-ups, exercise, and other self-care, as well as routine examinations such as mammograms, colonoscopies, and lab tests. We desperately need to develop preventive tools for mental health that are at least as effective as those we have for physical health.

There are strong forces at work against taking a health approach versus an illness approach to how we deliver care for both mental health and physical health. Among these forces are the profiteers masquerading as so-called "managed care" companies. There have been plenty of horror stories about victims of "mangled care" (which, in my opinion, is a more accurate description of so-called managed care). There have also been plenty of exposés about the corrupt practices of large health care companies. So many people are fed up with the mangled care companies that, when a young man assassinated the CEO of the largest such company (UnitedHealth Group) in December 2024, there was a tremendous amount of public support for the assassin. In April of 2025, CNN reported that his defense fund had so far raised $950,000 from 27,000 donors.[22]

.....I KNOW KA-RAZY.... REJECTING THE CAPITALIST ROAD TO TWISTED MENTAL HEALTH

The same corporations who control the quality and quantity of medical care provided in the U.S. also control the quality and quantity of mental health care provided. The U.S. spends more per person on health care than any other country,[23] yet ranks #69 on quality of care received.[24] In comparison, Cuba, a relatively poor nation that has been enduring an economic embargo perpetrated by the U.S. for several decades, ranks #27 in quality of health care. This situation is a result of the history of health care in the U.S.—a history shaped by profit-driven systems, fragmented delivery models, and decades of policy choices that have prioritized corporate interests over public wellbeing.

Our species, *Homo sapiens*, is said to have emerged 550,000 to 750,000 years ago in Africa.[25] It would make sense then that in all of those thousands of years, humans developed a lot of knowledge about medicine, if only through trial and error. As with other fields of human knowledge, the history of medicine is not usually recognized until it relates to Europe. All the scientific knowledge prior to that is often viewed through a racist lens as mysticism, voodoo, or witchcraft. My point is that it does not make sense to assume that only the knowledge accumulated over the last 200 years or so in Europe is what matters. Nevertheless, that is still the primary foundation of so-called modern health care.

Interestingly, even within the history of European-oriented medical knowledge, there were competing factions, and apparently the one that became dominant was not necessarily the better one. In the first half of the nineteenth century, the primary type of medicine was homeopathy. This approach was inspired by traditional non-European medicine in that it relied on the smallest possible doses of natural medicines. Homeopathy came to the U.S. in 1825, and in 1844 homeopathic medical doctors established the first professional medical association. The competing faction, the allopathic medical doctors, started the American Medical Association two years later, in 1846.[26] The difference between the two approaches seemed to be that homeopathy ("treatment by similars") was based on the idea that natural substances causing symptoms similar to a disease could be used to treat that disease, while allopathy ("treatment by opposites") relied on remedies that produced effects contrary to the symptoms—which at the time included methods such as blood-letting, crude forms of surgery, and the injection of toxic metals into the body.

Author E. Richard Brown, among others, has documented how the Rockefeller and Carnegie foundations, along with the American Medical Association (AMA), decided in the early twentieth century to take control of medical education in the U.S. Andrew Carnegie had made a fortune investing in steel, railroads, and oil, while John D. Rockefeller made a huge fortune by monopolizing the oil industry in the U.S. The AMA's Council on Medical Education approached the Carnegie Foundation to do a study of medical education.[27] The foundation hired a contractor named Abraham Flexner to create a report which was submitted to Congress in 1910. Flexner was not a medical professional or researcher, but he had Carnegie money backing him. He also garnered much of his information from the AMA. The Flexner report claimed, "there were too many doctors and medical schools in America, and that all the natural healing modalities which had existed for hundreds of years were unscientific quackery." Congress acted on this report and created laws making allopathic medicine the standard for medical practice and education.[28] Homeopathy and natural medicines were denounced, and the Rockefeller and Carnegie foundations used the power of their grants to medical schools to remove any discussion of diet and natural medicines from the curriculum. The same forces caused the closure of medical schools that would not comply with this approach. As a result, the number of medical schools in the U.S. went from 166 in 1904 to 76 in 1930. The AMA, along with other organizations promoting allopathic medicine, continued to dominate medical practice in the U.S. from the early twentieth century to the present.

Ironically, the precursor to managed care was a trend whose goals were the opposite of what managed care has become today. Starting in 1929 in Elk City, Oklahoma, and later in 1934 in Los Angeles, some medical doctors formed cooperatives intended to provide medical care to communities or groups of workers who paid an annual fee to receive care.²⁹ These cooperatives came to be called Health Maintenance Organizations in that their goals were to promote good health and prevent illness. These early forms of HMOs were denounced by the medical establishment but gained large numbers of enrollees.

Skipping ahead to the early 1970s, we find Democrat Ted Kennedy advocating for single-payer, universal health care while, on the Republican side, Richard Nixon was meeting with Edgar Kaiser of Kaiser Permanente, where he uttered this famous quote:

> Edgar Kaiser is running his Permanente deal for profit. And the reason that he can...the reason he can do it... I had Edgar Kaiser come in... talk to me about this and I went into it in some depth. All the incentives are toward less medical care, because... the less care they give them, the more money they make.³⁰

In 1973, Congress passed the Health Maintenance Organization Act and it was signed into law. But its goal was not to promote health—its goal was to control health care costs. This legislation introduced the concept of for-profit health care corporations in an industry that was mostly composed of non-profits. From there, for-profit managed care grew in the 1980s and 1990s. Now in 2025, we read about scandals involving how managed care has taken over Medicare (government funded medical care for senior citizens) through so-called "Medicare Advantage Plans."

Managed care companies are now large enough to bribe politicians, lobby them, and work to prevent the passage of legislation that could allow the U.S. to at least catch up with other developed capitalist countries who have been providing universal health care for decades.

Already bad at providing medical care, for-profit U.S. health care corporations have been equally bad at providing mental health care. It was not until 2008 that a new federal law required insurance companies to provide coverage for mental health issues equal to the coverage provided for medical issues. However, even 12 years later, there remained plenty of disparity, including the fact that the law does not require parity in reimbursement rates. Reimbursement rates are the fees paid directly to providers or reimbursed to patients who have already paid their providers.

According to NAMI (the National Alliance on Mental Illness, a major advocacy group for families of people who suffer from mental illness), people "cannot find in-network mental health care providers."[31] This means that a person might have to pay significantly more to see a so-called out-of-network provider. And often the out-of-network provider cannot get paid by the insurance company at all, so the member becomes liable for the entire fee for every session. For most people, the cost is prohibitive, especially since there are few if any mental health issues that can be properly addressed in just two or three sessions.

Additionally, the 2008 parity law carries no enforcement provisions other than having consumers wade through complex state and federal regulations to make individual complaints. And in 2025, there are indications the Trump administration is supporting a lawsuit by large employers to roll-back the parity law.[32] The large employers claim the parity law makes it difficult for them to provide affordable health care coverage to their employees. This is an Orwellian notion suggesting that health care can be made more affordable by stripping away the very coverage people need most (as NAMI puts it, "there is no health care without mental health care").

This argument by employers also provides yet another reason to take health care coverage out of the hands of employers. There are simply too many people who stay at jobs they hate, primarily because they need to keep health care coverage for themselves or a loved one with a chronic health condition.

By denying coverage to people who are unemployed, denying payment for certain kinds of treatment even to those who have coverage, and by effectively limiting coverage to illness rather than prevention, the capitalist system makes it clear it is not interested in promoting health but in cutting costs in order to increase profit. Many mangled care companies pay lip-service to the idea of prevention, but in practice they do not cover any preventive care unless the provider happens to bill it under one or two specific billing codes that the insurance company chooses to cover. And of course, knowing which billing code is likely to be covered is difficult for the provider to know, except by trial and denial. No wonder all the major stakeholders except the big capitalists hate mangled care. This includes consumers, providers, and a large portion of health care policy advocates including the American Public Health Association.

We can further assess the state of mental health under capitalism by looking more closely at the mental health of physicians, the professionals we rely on to treat our mental health. The suicide rate among physicians is significantly higher than that of the general population (which is already high). Moreover, the rate of suicide among physicians has been steadily increasing, and it shot up even higher during the COVID-19 pandemic.[33] While there are numerous contributing factors, the "system" has not been able to reduce the suicide rate among doctors. The biggest contributing factor is the "culture" taught and encouraged in medical schools. Amazingly, this culture promotes self-reliance and stigmatizes seeking mental health support among people who are supposed to encourage others to seek help.

Most people think of physicians as making a lot of money and living a good life. But the reality is quite different. A recent study shows that more than one third of physicians are considering leaving their profession. Two major reasons are burnout and too much administrative work. In particular, doctors get frustrated having to seek prior authorization (PA) from a clerk at an insurance company who has never seen or spoken to the patient. A physician-penned 2025 article reports that doctors generate about 40 PAs per week which require 13 hours to complete.[34] In a sure sign of the times, recent reports indicate that some major insurance companies are using artificial intelligence to automatically deny authorization for medical care.[35] One researcher reports that more than 850 million denials are issued each year, with only 1% appealed.[36] Let us keep in mind that these denials may frustrate physicians but ultimately the person who suffers the most is the individual whose care was denied.

To properly illustrate the nightmare some people go through, let's look at a few cases. One such case is that of John Samuel Maurer who began showing signs of schizophrenia in college. He was described as intelligent, charming, and handsome. One of his brothers was a psychiatrist and chief of staff at a state hospital, and one of his sisters was at one point the Los Angeles Mayor's deputy in charge of addressing homelessness. In spite of these connections, John ended up in the vicious cycle of criminal convictions (17), involuntary psych holds (too

.....I KNOW KA-RAZY.... REJECTING THE CAPITALIST ROAD TO TWISTED MENTAL HEALTH

many to count), six competency hearings, and one failed conservatorship.[37] His criminal convictions included "indecent exposure" and "discharge of a noxious substance" (most likely feces). A couple of his arrests resulted in competency hearings. Those hearings use the same narrow criteria as the ones the law requires to recognize someone as too insane to realize they were committing a crime. John was found competent to stand trial twice. The one time that he was determined to be incompetent he was referred for state-funded psychiatric treatment. However, the waiting list for such treatment had over 800 names ahead of him and he never made it to the top of the waiting list. In California, as in many other states, the one legal status that allows a person to be forced into treatment is a conservatorship. John was approved for a conservatorship, but apparently the law requires the conservatorship to be renewed annually. The renewal requires that a psychiatrist spend several hours in a court that is always running behind schedule waiting for a particular hearing to come up, so they can tell the court that a particular individual needs to continue under conservatorship. In John's case the psychiatrist did not show up, so his conservatorship was terminated. Ultimately, John's sister was approved as his conservator, but he remained in jail because his sister could not find an inpatient psych facility that was within driving distance and that would accept him in spite of his long and troubled history.

Another case involved Muhammad Shabazz Ali who lived in Dayton, Ohio. Muhammad had a severe mental illness and knew he needed to stay on medications, including anti-psychotic and anti-depressant prescriptions. He apparently ran out of medication and showed up at a facility very agitated, throwing chairs, hallucinating, and demanding, "I want my medications. I want my medications." The police were called and they transported him to a different psych facility. Even though the police had found him to be a grave danger to himself and others, that facility let him leave. Later that day, he shot three people and was charged with multiple counts of aggravated murder.[38] In March of 2018, he was convicted and given three life sentences plus 20 years without possibility of parole. Even though he was considered indigent, he was ordered to pay $8,411.91 in restitution (apparently for the funeral of one of his victims). There was no mention of any mental health care required as part of his prison term.[39]

Another case in Hendersonville, North Carolina involved a 60-year-old mother who worked part time as a school psychologist. Her son started having suicidal episodes at the age of 10. She spent many years battling insurance companies, school districts, hospitals, and treatment facilities trying to get him adequate psychiatric care. When he turned 17, she found herself calling emergency services 14 times in less than a year because he was threatening her. Eventually she made the heart-

.....I KNOW KA-RAZY.... REJECTING THE CAPITALIST ROAD TO TWISTED MENTAL HEALTH

wrenching decision to give up her parental rights and be declared a "neglectful parent" who is "unable or unwilling to provide a safe home for the juvenile, or to comply with mental health recommendations."[40] This was the only way she could get government entities to pay for her son's care. When yet another hospital called her to come pick him up, she felt her only option was to refuse.

Sometimes what is considered progress under capitalism ends up producing dubious outcomes. In the 1960s, the State of California was a prominent practitioner of de-institutionalization. When Ronald Reagan became governor in 1967, he stepped up this effort. The idea was to move all but the most dangerous mental patients out of hospitals and into boarding care homes in communities. These boarding care homes were privately owned and operated entities (sometimes actual homes, converted garages, or motels) that would try to make a profit by accepting social security disability payments in return for housing, feeding, and dispensing medication to individuals who were formerly inpatients at psychiatric facilities. In some cases, several of these homes would be owned by one company, such as California's Beverly Enterprises, which owned 38 homes. It turned out that five members of Beverly Enterprises' board had ties to Reagan, and their Board Chairman was the Vice Chair for a Ronald Reagan fundraiser.[41] Many of these boarding care homes did not have to be licensed and were not regulated in any way. The idea was that residents would receive treatment at some licensed outpatient facility while the boarding care homes served as housing. These homes had an incentive to provide the cheapest possible housing and food in order to try to make a profit from the $35 per day they were receiving per resident.

One individual who ended up spending 24 years in unlicensed boarding care homes was Eugene Walker of Los Angeles, California. Eugene was from an upper-middle-class African American family, and his father was a medical doctor. Eugene entered Yale University at age 17 and soon started showing signs of schizophrenia. He left college within a few months and after 10 years of cycling in and out of mental hospitals, he ended up in a boarding care home. At first his father was paying extra for somewhat better care, but eventually Eugene's care became dependent on his SSI check. The quality of care was poor, and patients were sometimes moved around to different homes—which in Eugene's case ranged from a garage in one community on the West Side of LA to a cottage in Compton. Thanks to his sister and her daughter, Eugene was finally liberated from the boarding care home "maze" and connected with both an effective outpatient treatment program and a proper nursing home. He went on to enroll in a community college, and at the age of 60, he was actively pursuing a bachelor's degree. (As sad as it may seem, Eugene's story is likely considered a success story under capitalist mental health care.)

.....I KNOW KA-RAZY.... REJECTING THE CAPITALIST ROAD TO TWISTED MENTAL HEALTH

If we were to consider the "other side" of the argument—that capitalist mental health care has helped many people, some with schizophrenia and others with less severe disorders, live productive lives—such a statement would be true overall. However, the main point is that capitalist health care started with a philosophically flawed approach. And once the powers that be began making billions using this flawed approach, they continued down the same path, even if it represented a twisted means for providing health care.

In 2011, Thomas Insell, director of the National Institute of Menta Health from 2002 to 2015, said, "Whatever we've been doing for five decades, it ain't working. When I look at the numbers—the number of suicides, the number of disabilities, the mortality data—it's abysmal, and it's not getting any better."[42]

Author Bruce E. Levine points out that,

> Researchers have long known that any single antidepressant drug is little more effective than a placebo in the majority of trials, shown to be less effective than a placebo in some studies, and generally found to be "clinically negligible" with respect to depression remission, while often resulting in severe adverse effects; for example, resulting in a higher percentage of sexual dysfunction than depression remission. However, for nearly twenty years, psychiatry and Big Pharma have told us that while one antidepressant may not work for the majority of patients, in the "real world," doctors provide patients who have been failed by their initial antidepressant with another antidepressant, and if that fails, still another; and that this real-world treatment is successful for nearly 70% of patients.[43]

Levine goes on to point out that this alleged 70% success rate is the result of a flawed study that some researchers found to be fraudulent. The only understandable motive for this kind of unethical—if not outright criminal—behavior is revealed by the astronomical amounts of money generated by these ineffective drugs. Just one drug, Zyprexa, dealt by Eli Lilly and used to treat schizophrenia and bipolar disorder, is reported to have earned the dealer $60.6 billion by 2017. In 2017, Eli Lilly was sued by the U.S. Department of Justice for failing to disclose that they had known the drug caused diabetes and other metabolic disorders. The dealer paid $1.4 billion to settle the suit. They saw it as a cost of doing business.[44]

Levine believes this kind of health care persists because of what he calls the "psychiatric-pharmaceutical-industrial complex." Big Pharma is able to spread some of its huge profits around to professional institutions such as the American Psychiatric Association, and even to so-called "patient advocacy" groups like NAMI. Big Pharma even paid $1.6 million in consulting fees to Harvard psychiatrist Joseph Biederman, who is credited with "inventing" pediatric bipolar disorder. This kind of invented diagnosis represents a potential gold mine for drug companies eager to medicate children for life.

Payments such as those to Biederman were not discovered until congress passed a law in 2013 requiring the disclosure of such transactions. The legislation resulted in disclosure that, from 2014 to 2020, "pharmaceutical companies paid $340 million to U.S. psychiatrists to serve as their consultants, advisers, and speakers, or to provide free food, beverages, and lodging to those attending promotional events."[45] Further, by 2019, Big Pharma was reportedly spending $6.6 billion per year on TV advertising, making them the fourth largest spender on TV ads in the U.S. This helps explain all the commercials urging us to ask our doctors about this or that miracle drug—each one promising relief from the horrors of yet another recently discovered disorder, such as "restless leg syndrome."

Another aspect of the psychiatric-pharmaceutical-industrial complex is that Big Pharma hires former officials from government agencies responsible for drug approval, enabling them to better communicate with former colleagues when submitting the next drug for approval. This psychiatric-pharmaceutical-industrial complex seems to work in ways that are remarkably similar to the military-industrial complex. One could make an argument that this kind of collusion is corrupt. But it's not so important "what" we call it. What matters is that we recognize that it does not operate to serve the best interests of the people who consume this kind of drug-centered health care.

Before we leave the topic of mangled care, it might be interesting to consider what options rich people have when it comes to health care. A quick internet search offers a glimpse:

- Dr. Jordan Shlain started a business called "Private Medical" with offices in San Francisco, Silicon Valley, Beverly Hills, Santa Monica, New York, and Miami. For $40,000 a year, clients gain access to a team consisting of 135 physicians, nurses, pharmacists, and medical support professionals around the clock. Home visits are provided as needed, and the annual fee covers office visits and tests. Hospitalizations are billed separately. Private Medical reportedly caters to individuals worth $100 million or more, and the business is projected to generate $11 billion in annual revenue by 2032.[46]

- Privé-Swiss is a mental health retreat that promises psychotherapy, meditation, a functional medicine nutritionist, massages, gourmet chef, customized facials, a car to take you out as needed along with a companion, and other aesthetic and holistic services. Their website says the duration of the treatment is customizable. There is no mention of accepting insurance, and of course, it's one of those places where if you need to know the cost in advance, you probably cannot afford it.[47]

- One Master's-level psychotherapist in New York City offers his services through a somewhat gimmicky "walk and talk" package.[48] Clients pay him $450 for a 50-minute session, and he takes them on a walk through Central Park as they talk. Interestingly, he considers himself on the more affordable end of NYC therapists, noting that others charge $1,000 for 45-minute sessions—and of course they don't accept insurance.

Wealthy individuals, it seems, have a lot of sweet options when it comes to mental health care. They do not have to be bothered with the health insurance headaches and nonsense the working class is forced to deal with.

CHAPTER 3

COPING STRATEGIES

BERNARD NICOLAS

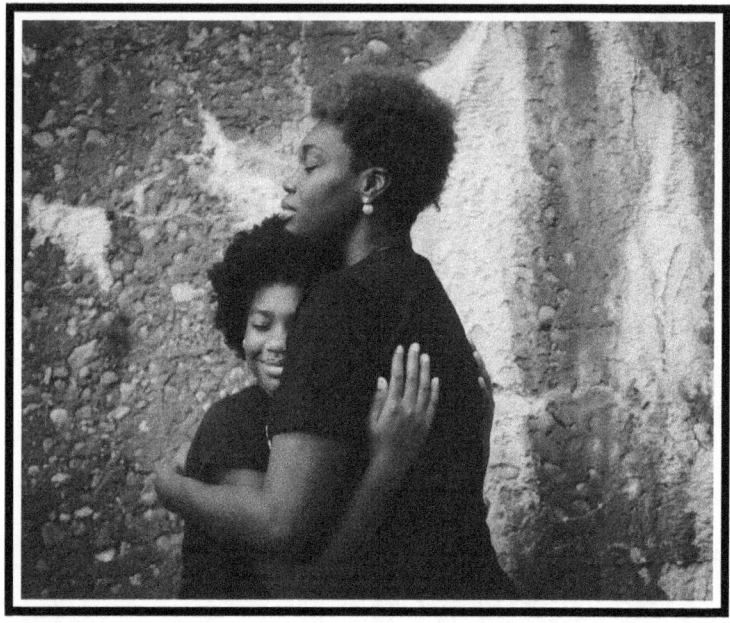

> Some just went "off" because it was the best "conscious, rational" thing they could think of at the time.

The *Penguin Dictionary of Psychology* defines coping strategies as "conscious, rational ways of dealing with the anxieties of life."[49] Unfortunately, when most people are looking for coping strategies, they are not feeling particularly rational. Thus, a more practical definition of coping would be "getting through the moment(s) by

.....I KNOW KA-RAZY.... REJECTING THE CAPITALIST ROAD TO TWISTED MENTAL HEALTH

seeking healthy or unhealthy ways of reducing the unbearable emotional pain."

To better understand coping strategies within the "ka-razy" context of dying capitalism, it helps to examine how people in various types of situations have tried to cope, and how some just went "off" because it was the best "conscious, rational" thing they could think of at the time.

Since we all have issues—and most of us do not have adequate access to quality mental health support—it follows that many of us turn to unhealthy coping mechanisms. Children who suffer severe abuse may develop one or more alternate personalities—a form of dissociative personality disorder—because they are unable to cope with the impact of the abuse on their original personality. Many people who are ultimately diagnosed with addiction to alcohol or another substance (a mental disorder) start out using that substance as a coping mechanism. Families and sometimes entire cultural groups use food as a coping mechanism. It is no coincidence that 40% of adults in the U.S. are officially classified as obese.

While the common belief is that widespread obesity in the U.S. stems from lack of exercise, recent research confirms that the primary cause is an unhealthy diet—particularly the consumption of highly processed foods.[50] Since heart disease, diabetes and strokes are in the top five leading causes of death in the U.S., and since diet is a major factor in all of these chronic conditions, one could argue that food kills more people than all illegal drugs put together. Overall, it seems that far more people use unhealthy coping mechanisms than healthy ones. Although the percentage of people seeking mental health services is increasing, most in the U.S. have never been exposed to the concept of mental health "self-care"—many have never even considered it an option.

Throughout history, there have been individuals who took radical action as a way of coping with severe conditions of oppression. In their book *Crazy as Hell*, authors Hoke Glover and Efua Prince call attention to a number of such individuals. In their foreword to the book, the authors state, "every enslaved person who dreamt of freedom dreamt an original crazy as hell thought."[51] The authors go on to point out that "slave ships were hell with sails—full of sickness, filth, rape, and shackles."[52] They then posit that it is difficult to say who was crazier, the people who chose to jump off the boat and die, or those who stayed on the boat hoping that things would get better once they got off. The enslavement of Africans was one of the greatest holocausts in the history of the planet. We will discuss below the psychology of resistance. But for now, the point is that most human beings try to accommodate and adapt, even under the most horrible conditions. But some of us get fed up with trying to "go along to get along" and just "go off."

There have been a number of movies that illustrate cases of people going off. No doubt, the attraction of

.....I KNOW KA-RAZY.... REJECTING THE CAPITALIST ROAD TO TWISTED MENTAL HEALTH

such movies comes from the sense of tremendous powerlessness that a lot of us feel. Living vicariously through the people who go off provides a momentary sense of relief. Denzel Washington's follow-up role after winning the Best Actor Academy Award for *Training Day* was in the film *John Q*, directed by Nick Cassavetes. John Q was a working-class guy unable to get a heart transplant for his son because of the limitations of mangled care (see previous chapter). John eventually goes off and takes a few people in the ER hostage. In the end, the film shows that most people support John Q and denounce the mangled care system. John Q clearly qualified for the "crazy as hell" or ka-razy label.

But sometimes people who qualify as ka-razy carry out actions that really frighten the system. The system then feels it has to kill those individuals to solve the problem. Clearly, the system's decision makers are not mentally healthy if they believe killing someone is more beneficial than trying to understand the conditions that led to the crimes committed by these ka-razies. No wonder the number of mass shootings in the U.S. just keeps increasing!

There are lessons to be learned by considering the circumstances of two individuals. These individuals are far removed from the stereotype of the typical mass shooter in that they were both African-American veterans. Let us consider John Allen Muhammad and Christopher Dorner.

John Allen Muhammad served 16 years in three different military organizations, one immediately after the other. These were the Louisiana National Guard, the U.S. Army, and then the Oregon National Guard. During his more than eight years in the U.S. Army, John Allen trained as a sniper and served in the 1991 Gulf War. Over several years, John Allen was involved in an intense battle with his ex-wife regarding custody of their three children. John Allen's best friend Robert Holmes, who had known him since 1985 said that for John Allen...

> I think that after his kids got taken away John had a nervous breakdown. I'm not a professor or a doctor, but John changed in a million subtle ways after his kids were taken away. He'd spend all day some days just crying. All he could think of was getting his kids back.[53]

Both Robert and John Allen's divorce lawyer, John Mills, indicated that failure to get even partial custody of his children was the event that pushed John Allen over the edge. His devotion to fatherhood had even led him to informally adopt the teenage son of a divorced Jamaican mother. This adopted son was Lee Boyd Malvo. John taught Lee Boyd how to shoot a rifle, just as he had taught his other son. John Allen and Lee Boyd Malvo

.....I KNOW KA-RAZY.... REJECTING THE CAPITALIST ROAD TO TWISTED MENTAL HEALTH

became infamous when they went on a sniping spree across the U.S. and killed 17 people across 10 states. John Allen was executed in Virginia in half the time it normally takes to execute people who are sentenced to death. The mainstream media treated the execution as a "problem solved," no further discussion required. Imagine if, instead of receiving the death penalty, John Allen had been required to agree to be interviewed by an unlimited number of serious researchers seeking to understand aspects of his life in exchange for a life sentence. In a capitalist culture where uncovering problems is likely to mean money will have to be spent, it is much cheaper to kill someone than to learn from that person. In John Allen's background, there were several instances where a more effective intervention could have changed the trajectory of his life. These instances include more sensible psychological considerations when a person is trained in the military to see humans as targets to be eliminated without hesitation or remorse. They also include the situations that led to John Allen striking his sergeant in the head, being sentenced to seven days in the stockade, and then having his sentence suspended. John Allen reportedly had learning disabilities in school and was clearly extremely depressed when he could not get even partial custody of his children. Yet, never in his life was he referred for a psychological evaluation. When the army teaches snipers to overcome the natural human resistance to murder another human, do they try to counteract this training upon discharge from the Army? Not likely—and it's even less likely that the training of a sniper can be undone.

The judicial system was eager to convict and kill John Allen Muhammad, not only because he had killed innocent people, but also because his sniper spree exposed how easily one man and a teenager hiding in the trunk of a Chevy Caprice could terrorize an entire country for days. One might hope that executing him was meant to serve as a deterrent to others who might take similar paths to the extremes of ka-razy—but since John Allen's execution, the U.S. has witnessed thousands of mass shooting incidents. When an individual's mental health condition drives that person to cope with real or perceived injustice in extreme ways, it is highly unlikely that logical thinking about possible punishment ever enters into the equation.

The case of **Christopher Jordan Dorner** is another example of an individual with no history of diagnosed mental health issues who took extreme measures to relieve perceived injustice. Interestingly, his case exposes not only his mental health, but that of the individual Dorner tried to expose for mistreating a mentally ill citizen, as well as the dangerous paranoia of police officers who were looking for Dorner after he had killed several people, including the niece of an LAPD captain.

Christopher Dorner was born in California's Orange County and wanted to be a police officer from a very

.....I KNOW KA-RAZY.... REJECTING THE CAPITALIST ROAD TO TWISTED MENTAL HEALTH

young age. He was very excited to be admitted to the LAPD training academy. His training there was interrupted because he was in the U.S. Navy reserve and was deployed overseas for 13 months. After some difficulties, he eventually completed his academy course of study. His training officer on patrol was a woman named Teresa Evans. Dorner reported that he witnessed Evans kicking a handcuffed, mentally ill man in the face and collar bone because the man was being uncooperative. Dorner further reported that his training officer, along with another Sergeant, persuaded him not to include the kicks in his arrest report. Dorner later filed a complaint against Evans who, according to him, had a reputation of past abusive acts and was "an angry woman" who felt wronged by both her active-duty LAPD officer boyfriend and her ex-husband, a former-LAPD officer. A hearing was held, and Dorner was accused of making up the kicking part of the incident and was fired from the LAPD in December 2008. In February 2013, little more than four years later, Dorner was accused of killing the daughter of a retired LAPD captain and her fiancé. Ironically, this retired captain was the lawyer who represented Dorner at his hearing after the complaint about Evans.

Dorner posted an 11,000-word manifesto online in which he admitted killing the captain's daughter and claimed that the purpose of his actions was to clear his name which had been sullied by the racism inherent at the LAPD. He was aware that he might not be alive at the end of his crusade, but he listed a number of targets that he intended to eliminate, nonetheless. Donner mentioned in his manifesto that it should not have been so easy for him to obtain the small arms that he was using in his campaign. He praised President Obama's accomplishments but also remembered a great friend who once told him that no matter how much he accomplished in life he would always be a nigger in the eyes of many. He also wrote that some friends told him he should have kept quiet instead of making a complaint about a fellow officer. His response to those friends was, "maybe you were right. But I'm not built like others, it's not in my DNA, and my history has always shown that."[54] In other words, it was not in Dorner's nature to keep quiet when faced with unethical behavior. His manifesto went on to praise a variety of celebrities and stand up for LGBTQ rights. Dorner ended by writing that "Blacks must strive for more in life than bling, hoes, and cars. The current culture is an epidemic that leaves them with no discernable future." (Thus, the ka-razy guy comments on the craziness of the culture!)

Nothing in his manifesto explained how Dorner's thinking may have progressed during the four years between his firing from LAPD and the start of his killing spree. Most likely he was obsessing over the injustice he felt had been done to him and he eventually developed a compulsive plan to get revenge. His manifesto did not suggest he would ever simply make up a false accusation against a fellow police officer as was alleged. So, it's most likely he felt genuinely wronged by the LAPD—a possibility reinforced when, subsequent to Dorner's murderous actions, other Black former LAPD officers spoke out in support of his denunciation of racism at the LAPD.[55] To give a sense of the racial climate within the LAPD at the time, a 2008 ACLU report found that the Black stop rate—defined as LAPD officers pulling over Black people—was 3,400 stops higher per 10,000 residents than the white stop rate.[56] Years before, perhaps the most influential chief of the LAPD, William Parker, appeared before the U.S. Commission on Civil Rights in 1960 and said, "The established community thinks cops are not hard enough on Blacks." In a TV interview in the same year he made the following remark,

> It is estimated that by 1970, 45 percent of the metropolitan area of Los Angeles will be Negro. If you want any protection for your home... you're going to have to get in and support a strong police department. If you don't, come 1970, God help you.[57]

The headquarters of the LAPD bore the name of William Parker for 53 years. Parker's driver, Darryl Gates, was the serving LAPD chief when Rodney King was brutally beaten by LAPD officers.

Dorner's actions resulted in a huge manhunt and a massive effort to protect potential targets mentioned by Dorner in his manifesto. Officers protecting one such target opened fire on a truck that was driven by two Latinas who were delivering newspapers. The officers fired 107 bullets before realizing that the women were not Dorner and looked nothing like him. None of the officers who fired were found to have misbehaved.

Many years after Dorner's suicide by cop, particularly during the era of the George Floyd protests, Dorner was elevated by some people to folk-hero status for daring to take on the LAPD.[58] Clearly Dorner was far from mentally healthy. But then neither was officer Evans or the officers who fired 107 bullets at unarmed innocent women. Often when police officers abuse their authority and hurt or kill citizens, the "bad apple" argument takes over. This argument seeks to sustain the fallacy that the murder of innocent citizens is caused by isolated bad apple officers. The notion that the entire police culture might have a serious problem is usually attacked by representatives of the ruling system, while those advocating for systemic reform are often labeled as crazy extremists. Perhaps, as the authors of *Crazy as Hell* indicate in their foreword, "This whole country is crazy as hell."[59]

Given that many people find themselves cornered by impossible conditions of oppression, it is not possible to

.....I KNOW KA-RAZY.... REJECTING THE CAPITALIST ROAD TO TWISTED MENTAL HEALTH

fully understand ka-razy as a coping mechanism without looking at the psychology of resistance. In 2025, we have several decades of anti-colonial struggle to consider, even as the Palestinian people in Gaza are actively suffering from a genocide perpetrated by settler colonialism, rationalized by Zionist ideas. Writing in support of the Palestinian struggle, Adnan Hmidan points out that "liberation has never been won by petitions or carefully phrased condemnations. Algerians did not wait for national consensus before rising up against French colonial rule. The Vietnamese didn't call roundtable meetings before confronting U.S. military occupation."[60]

Perhaps the greatest contributor to the psychology of resistance, Frantz Fanon was a psychiatrist from Martinique who ended up working in Algeria during the anti-colonial struggle. His observations about the impact of colonialism and of the struggle against it inspired him to write several seminal books and to become an active member of the Algerian Liberation Front.

Referring to Fanon's first major work, *Black Skins, White Mask*, a Turkish PhD student wrote in 2025, "Here, he argues that colonialism constructs the Black and the white, such that to be healthy is to be white, producing 'aberrations of affect' among Black people as 'health' would demand they pursue an unachievable whiteness."[61] Another student of Fanon pointed out that Fanon "saw how colonial psychiatry naturalized mental disorders that were in fact determined by social and cultural factors."[62]

The dying capitalist system does the same thing these observers mentioned. Directly and indirectly (particularly through imagery) they define good mental health as earning a good income through persistent effort and living a life enhanced by the possession of the right clothes, car, and a happy pet. For those who burn out while trying to achieve this unachievable whiteness, the system has institutions, therapy groups, and drugs that encourage people to take responsibility for their situations, never acknowledging the power of the economic and political conditions that created the mental disorder.

Louise Little was born as a result of the rape of her then 11-year-old mother. Her husband Earl Little "was brutally murdered because he was an activist for social justice. After his death, she was left to raise 10 children on her own."[63] It should not surprise anyone that Louise Little ended up locked up in a psychiatric hospital in Kalamazoo, Michigan for 25 years. She was only released when her son— who came to be known as Malcom X—joined with his brothers to secure her release. Like Louise Little, there are thousands of individuals today who are effectively 100% psychologically disabled because they simply could not make sense of desperately trying and failing to achieve that unachievable whiteness.

.....I KNOW KA-RAZY.... REJECTING THE CAPITALIST ROAD TO TWISTED MENTAL HEALTH

On January 1, 2025, Shamsud-Din Jabbar drove a pickup truck through a crowded street in New Orleans and killed 14 people. On the same day, Matthew Livelsberger, blew himself up in a Tesla truck in front of the Trump Hotel in Las Vegas. Both of these men were veterans. One was African American and the other was a white American. No doubt they both had serious mental health issues. These incidents inspired Professor Juan Cole to write a piece listing the top 10 differences between white Terrorists and others. Item #2 on his list reads, "White terrorists are 'troubled loners.' Other terrorists are always suspected of being part of a global plot, even when they are obviously troubled loners." Item #4 on his list points out that, "The family of a white terrorist is interviewed, weeping as they wonder where the person went wrong. The families of other terrorists are almost never interviewed."[64] In a piece done by *Forbes* about Livelsberger, his ex-girlfriend, Alicia Arritt, indicated that his behavior started changing in 2019 when he returned from deployment with a traumatic brain injury. She indicated that Livelsberger received no treatment for his PTSD because it's not "acceptable to seek treatment when someone is in special forces."[65] Shamsud-Din Jabbar was also an individual whose life was unraveling and who also received no mental health support. The fact that he placed an ISIS flag on his truck before his rampage allowed the major media to report his action as radical terrorism, even though the Associated Press could find no connection between him and any terrorist group. In fact, they quoted a friend of Shamsud—someone who had worked in military anti-terrorism—affirming that he had seen no red flags suggesting that his friend could ever commit an act like this.[66] The FBI confirmed soon after the rampage that Shamsud acted alone.[67]

In his recent book, *The Fort Bragg Cartel*, veteran Seth Harp points out the impact of multiple years of war on U.S. Special Forces soldiers:

> Behind a heavy curtain of government secrecy, twenty-plus years at war in Afghanistan, Iraq, Yemen, Libya, Somalia, Syria, the Philippines, and elsewhere has given rise in this ultra-elite unit to a toxic culture of addiction, criminality, madness, violence, and impunity.[68]

When people cannot cope, some see only suicide as the solution. Some people who complete a suicide choose to do so in a spectacular way that brings attention to issues they have apparently obsessed about. One could easily argue that all of the cases mentioned above, John Allen Muhammad, Christopher Dorner, Shamsud-Din Jabbar, and Matthew Livelsberger died by forms of suicide. It's also easy to conclude that the aspect of mental

..... I KNOW KA-RAZY.... REJECTING THE CAPITALIST ROAD TO TWISTED MENTAL HEALTH

health in each of these cases was not sufficiently investigated. Ironically, sometimes mental illness can be used as a method of dismissing any legitimate criticism an individual may have about our unhealthy culture.

Some scholars have argued that Ted Kaczynski, whom the FBI labeled the "Unabomber," was actually not as mentally ill as he was made out to be. He was actually a brilliant individual who was admitted to Harvard at age 16 and was granted a tenure track position at UC Berkeley at age 25, "the youngest such hire in the history of the University."[69] While, ultimately, he cannot be held up as an example of good mental health, we can view him instead as someone who had strong feelings and offered a detailed argument about his assessment that "the industrial revolution and its consequences have been a disaster for the human race."[70] Because Kaczynski committed violent acts that caused the death of others, politics demanded that he be marginalized as "insane." Kaczynski completed suicide in June 2023.[71]

Absent any constructive channel for investing thoughts and feelings that are highly critical of our current systems, and having no access to mental health support that does not seek to pathologize radical political criticism, we are likely to continue to experience cases of individuals who "go off" and commit murderous acts. The only way to prevent such incidents is to provide good mental health support and healthy coping strategies. This will be discussed later in chapter 10.

BERNARD NICOLAS

CONCEPTS OF MENTAL HEALTH

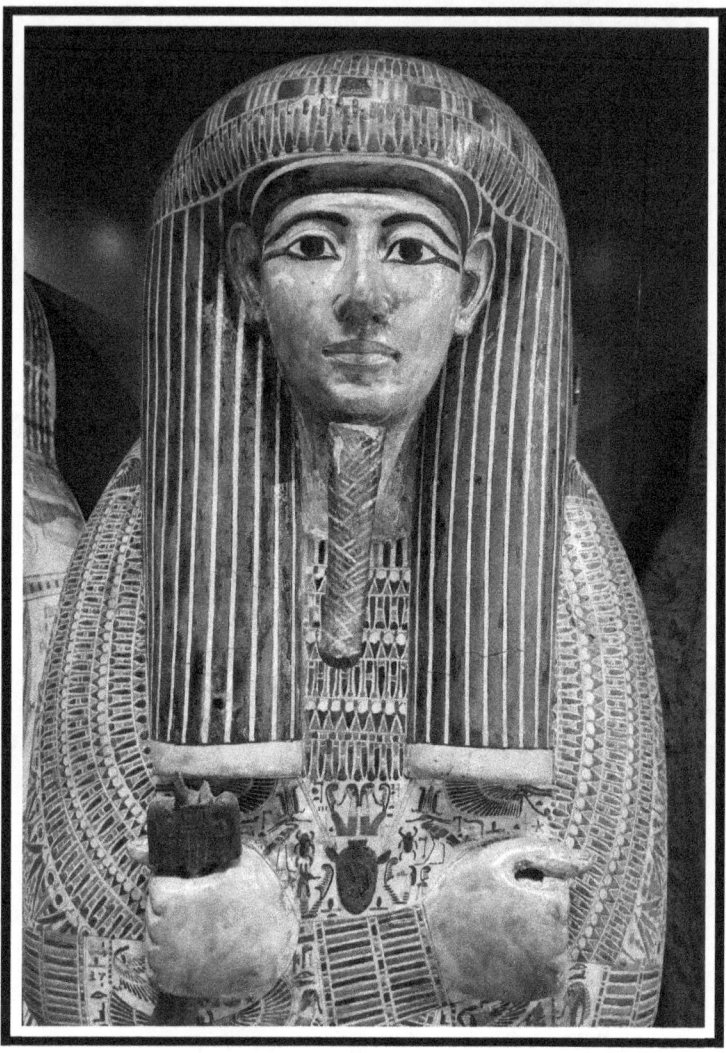

.....I KNOW KA-RAZY.... REJECTING THE CAPITALIST ROAD TO TWISTED MENTAL HEALTH

> When seeking health advice, it is best not to exclusively consult the most successful drug dealer in your community.

It is a common practice of individual and group self-deception to assume that whatever is being advocated by powerful people and institutions in the present is the most modern, most advanced level of thought that ever existed. Fortunately, many people today have come to understand that it makes a lot more sense to consider all of human history when searching for pearls of wisdom, rather than relying on the thoughts of people whose profit-driven motives are totally questionable. In other words, when seeking health advice, it is best not to exclusively consult the most successful drug dealer in your community. (In this context drug dealer refers to what has become the primary characteristic of so-called modern medicine and psychiatry, the large drug companies, aka Big Pharma.)

Throughout most of known human history, and particularly in cultures that thrived for many hundreds of years, concepts of health have been holistic and based on concepts of "being." As described by Wade W. Nobles, scholar of African Psychology, "Given ancient African thought, both Beingness and Becoming would be based on the principle of Ka or universal spirit. The fundamental basis of all things (whether as a state of being or in the process of becoming) is spirit or energy."[72] Nobles goes on to point out that...

> ... to be normal is to be consistent with the dictates of one's Ka... Attitudinally and behaviorally normal or natural functioning is represented by (1) a sense of self which is collective or extended; (2) and attitude wherein one understands and respects the sameness in oneself and others; (3) a clear sense of one's spiritual connection to the universe...[73]

Similarly, Turkish-American Jungian Psychologist Ipek S. Burnett posits that "personal is always political, and psychic distress and public struggles belong together."[74]

In an article entitled "Chinese Philosophy has long known that mental health is communal," Asian-American Studies professor Alexus McLeod quotes Dutch cultural psychologist Batja Mesquita who defines human emotions very differently from modern western psychology: "Many cultures don't think of their emotions as something that lives inside an individual, but more as something that lives between people. In those cultures, emotions are what people do together, with each other. So when I'm angry, that is something that lives between you and me."[75]

This well-founded notion of mental health as communal is consistent with the concept of mental health as a spectrum rather than a binary proposition, that one is either healthy or sick. Most of us know one of "those people" who are obviously "two cans short of a six-pack." We also know of people who were considered brilliant right up to the moment they were discovered to have been severely mentally ill all along. This was the case with the brilliant mathematician John Nash, whose story was released in 2001 as a movie called *A Beautiful Mind*. Nash seemed to have unusual mental perceptions that allowed him to work on U.S. government contracts via the RAND Corporation. He is said to have been involved in breaking codes during the Cold War, and his contributions to game theory have been widely applied by business and government. When his symptoms became more obvious, he was found to be a paranoid schizophrenic. However, with professional help, he learned to manage his illness and was able to win a Nobel prize more than 30 years after he was first diagnosed.

Many successful businesspeople are actually psychopaths who are able to fire thousands of employees without remorse. According to forensic psychologist Robert Hare, a psychopath is four times more likely to be a CEO than a janitor.[76] A psychopath is someone who is often charming and intelligent but is pathologically egocentric and has no capacity to love. We tend to positively value people who make a lot of money, show high energy, and like to have a good time. Yet, none of these factors indicate good mental health.

We also tend to fear people who display "abnormal" behavior such as having auditory or visual delusions. Yet such people are usually far less dangerous than those who appear successful but are actually psychopaths or sociopaths. Many sociopaths are very dangerous, while others are high-functioning, attractive people who harm others emotionally whenever they are not busy boosting their ego by doing things for others. One sociopath has written a book about herself in which she states,

> I have never killed anyone, but I have certainly wanted to. I may have a disorder, but I am not crazy. In a world filled with mediocre nothings populating a go-nowhere rat race, people are attracted to my exceptionalism like moths to a flame.[77]

From the point of view described above, which considers individual mental health as communal and spiritual, the sociopath is the extreme other end of the mental health spectrum. What exactly causes some mental disorders such as schizophrenia or bipolar disorder is still unknown. Clearly some mental health issues are caused by family-of-origin-based trauma, often experienced in childhood, while others are impacted by broader forces known as the collective unconscious, intergenerational psychological trauma, or alienation.

A major theoretician on human psychology, Carl Jung, sought to explain why so many cultures have similar myths and stories. He came up with the notion of the "collective unconscious." This was a significant improvement on Sigmund Freud's idea that the unconscious was strictly a product of personal experiences.[78] The Jungian concept of the collective unconscious is compatible with the notion that mental health is communal and that emotions occur between people rather than inside individuals. The notion of intergenerational trauma explains that people who have suffered historical trauma pass on the impact of this trauma to their descendants through their genes as well as their behavior. Although some trauma victims may not talk about their experiences, everything about their behavior tells their kids that the world is not safe and horrible things can happen at any time. Dr. Joy DeGruy studied a particular kind of intergenerational trauma which she calls Post Traumatic Slavery Syndrome. DeGruy argues that people, such as descendants of African slavery victims, have experienced intergenerational trauma and developed survival mechanisms and other patterns of behavior that can have both negative and positive impacts. She points out that,

> As we heal we also have to move ahead. To do so we can build upon traditional strengths that we relied upon all along: our spirituality and faith, our sense of community, and our tradition of great leaders.[79]

As Dr. DeGruy implies, all victims of intergenerational trauma and oppression can build on their strengths collectively in order to heal. But before they can heal, they have to overcome the self-loathing that trauma can cause and realize that their problem is not an individual but a collective one.

The concept of alienation under capitalism can help us to understand the self-loathing of the oppressed. Alienation is, the sense of disconnection and estrangement that individuals often experience in capitalist societies. This concept goes beyond mere feelings of loneliness or isolation, delving into the profound psychological impact of being separated from the products of one's labor, from nature, from one's own human essence, and from other people.[80]

The alienated individual, like the victim of Post Traumatic Slavery Syndrome, can develop "learned helplessness, literacy deprivation, distorted self-concept, and antipathy or aversion for... the mores and customs associated with one's own identified cultural/ethnic heritage."[81] People who are alienated from themselves are prone to adopting values propagated by the very system that oppresses them. Usually, those values suggest that if an individual is not doing well it is probably because he/she is inferior, broken, or just not trying hard enough. They can also take up what Marx called "commodity fetishism." Commodity fetishism helps us to understand why in capitalist cultures, owning a particular brand-name commodity, such as an iPhone or a designer handbag or a Lamborghini, can become an obsession for certain individuals who mistakenly believe these commodities reflect who they are and their self-worth.

One powerful revelation about the level of alienation in the U.S. involves the declaration of an "epidemic of loneliness." This declaration was made in late Spring of 2023 by then Surgeon General of the U.S., Vivek Murthy. Murthy considered his declaration an urgent advisory and indicated that "loneliness is far more than just a 'bad feeling' and represents a major health risk for both individuals and society."[82] Harvard University's Graduate School of Education invested four years in a study of loneliness. They found that "people between 30-44 years of age were the loneliest group — 29% of people in this age range said they were 'frequently' or 'always' lonely."[83] In comparison, the 65-and-over age group only had 10% report being always or frequently lonely. The same study found that people earning under $30,000 per year had a 29% rate of frequent loneliness, compared to those earning over $100,000 with an 18% rate.[84] The Surgeon General's advisory reported that in 2018 only 16% of respondents felt very attached to their local community.[85] The advisory also admitted that while technology broadens our communities and opens the world to those with limited access, it also can "make us feel worse about ourselves and our relationships. Some technology fans the flames of discrimination, bullying, and other forms of social negativity."[86]

Popular social media platforms which now have billions of users were intentionally designed to foster behavioral addiction. The University of Michigan institute for Healthcare Policy reported that "Social media platforms are using the same techniques as gambling firms to create psychological dependencies and ingrain their products in the lives of their users... These methods are so effective that they can activate similar mechanisms as cocaine in the brain..."[87] The co-founder of Facebook, Sean Parker disclosed that Facebook is "a social validation feedback loop... exactly the kind of thing that a hacker like myself would come up with, because you're exploiting a vulnerability in human psychology... The inventors, creators understood this consciously. And we did it anyway."[88]

Social media has also been found to impact body image and depression.[89] Platforms that encourage posting and editing selfies, promote "fitspiration" content that idealizes thinness, or suggest an ideal body type are likely to aggravate body image issues. *Psychology Today* reported on a study of teens in Canada that showed improved appearance and weight esteem among youths who reduced their social media use to one hour per day.[90]

Clearly, technology also offers mental health benefits by making useful information and telehealth sessions more accessible. The main challenge is how to promote the beneficial aspects of technology while controlling the negative ones. In theory, laissez-faire capitalism prefers to let the market regulate all effects, positive or negative. The naïve theory is that if people don't want negative effects, they will not pay for them, and the product with the negative effects will disappear from the marketplace. But in current times, we often don't know about the negative effects and we are not the ones who pay for the product. As in the case of social media, using it is "free" because the paying customers are the entities that buy ads to put in our feeds. So, Facebook will not disappear from the market unless the company is no longer able to sell our information to advertisers.

If the completely idealistic notion of letting the market decide everything had any value, capitalism would have never developed the need for so much regulation and alleged redistribution of income via taxation. Besides its failure to implement free markets that manage themselves, capitalism has yet to develop a method for assigning value to mental health benefits and deficits that are difficult to quantify. Nevertheless, just by using metrics such as missed days at work and unemployment due to chronic illness, the Meharry School of Global Health was able to project that the cumulative cost of mental health inequities from 2024 to 2040 will add up to $14 trillion.[91]

In a system that prioritizes human wellbeing, no technology should be allowed to have more negative than positive impact. Thus, businesses that become so large that they risk impacting the wellbeing of most of the population would definitely need to be under management and ownership of their workers. And if this ownership and management was not enough to bring the business in line with system priorities, then some other form of community management would be necessary. Even under capitalism, some have suggested that social media companies should be nationalized.

> As we can control and decide over what happens on our streets, libraries, markets, schools and universities, we should be able to control and decide over what happens in our Newsfeeds, which algorithms apply to us and whether and which advertisements reach us. In this way we can make sure that the fabric of society does not unravel, that even its margins stay in contact with each other so that the public sphere remains intact. As part of the democratic public sphere, social media belongs into the hands of citizens.[92]

The only way to apply the concept that "being" and "mental health" have a collective dimension is to structure and manage everything that can affect our sense of being and our mental health in line with collective wellbeing as the #1 priority. While ancient Egyptians wanted us to have a clear sense of spiritual connection to the universe, advanced capitalism relegated us to a lonely and addictive attachment to devices that seem to enhance our sense of alienation from ourselves and others. It is not surprising then that public health under capitalism has failed to give proper regard to our mental health.

MENTAL HEALTH AS PUBLIC HEALTH

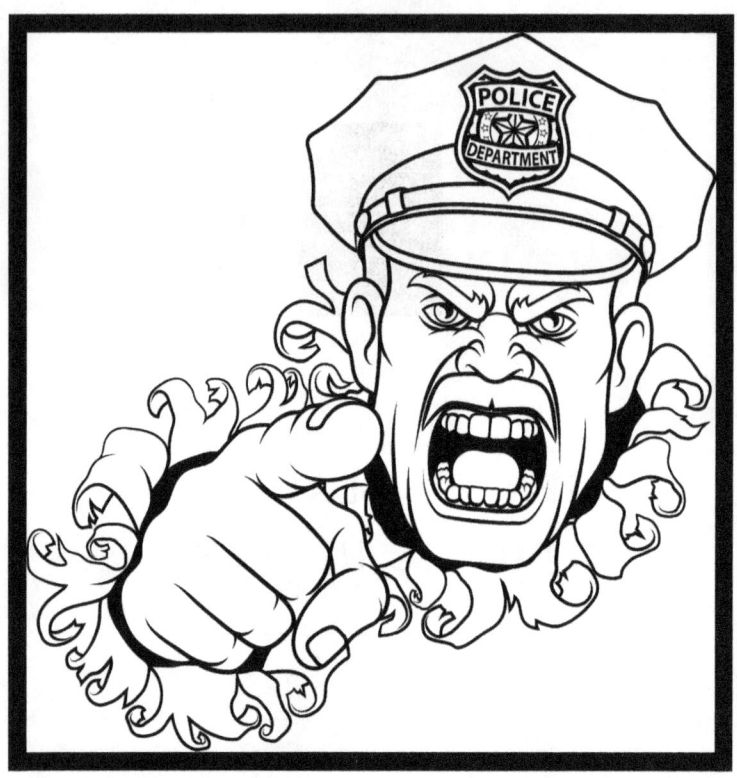

> Apparently, the police culture continues to discourage mental health maintenance due to the stigma associated with it—a stigma ironically similar to the one that plagues physicians.

According to the CDC, the percentage of adults counselled by mental health professionals in 2024 was 14%. When broken down by race, white adults accessed mental health services about twice as much as Black adults. Clearly the vast majority of the population does not access mental health counseling on a regular basis. Many individuals are prescribed psychotropic medications by their primary care doctors. Such doctors usually have no special training in psychology and likely base their prescriptions on brochures provided by the drug company. Nevertheless, such prescriptions are considered mental health "treatment."

According to an article published by Tulane university School of Public Health, "Mental health has a huge impact on how people relate to others, make decisions, and handle stress. People's ability to live fulfilling lives often depends on their mental health. This makes protecting and restoring mental health of immediate concern to public health professionals."[93] The same article also points out that "up to 75 percent of youth in the juvenile justice system who are disproportionately from racial and ethnic minorities have mental health disorders."[94]

For several decades, the Los Angeles County Jail system has been considered "the largest mental health facility in the United States."[95] According to *California Healthline*, "Across California and the U.S., far more people with mental illness are housed in jails and prisons than in psychiatric hospitals."[96] Although it seems like a nice idea to think about treating mentally unhealthy people in the community, the reality is that some severely mentally unhealthy individuals need more intense residential care. Writer Patrick Cockburn pointed out in 2017, that "between 1955 and 2016, the number of state hospital beds in the U.S. available to psychiatric patients fell by 97 percent from 559,000 to just 38,000."[97]

These facts alone are an indicator of the public health crisis we currently face relative to mental health. Many families, including middle-class families with a mentally ill member, have to endure the recurring trauma of watching their loved one repeat a cycle of jail, brief treatment, addiction, and back to jail. This vicious cycle is heartbreaking. Understandably, people in a so-called advanced society want to believe that any illness should be manageable with real treatment rather than jailhouse treatment.

Compared to the U.S., several countries are considered to promote better mental health. Contributing factors are "work-life balance, government health-care spending and environmental factors, including green spaces."[98] In June 2025, the U.S. Centers for Disease Control (CDC), under the Trump administration, was allowed to state the obvious:

.....I KNOW KA-RAZY.... REJECTING THE CAPITALIST ROAD TO TWISTED MENTAL HEALTH

> CDC's public health strategy to improve mental health is guided by principles of health equity. Health equity is the state in which everyone has a fair and just opportunity to attain their highest level of health. When people have limited access to the resources they need to stay healthy, such as access to health care, they are more likely to struggle with health issues.[99]

In the U.S., around 30 million people are estimated to have no health insurance. The "Affordable Care Act" under Obama increased the number of people with health insurance coverage. Huge differences continue to exist when access to health care for non-Hispanic whites is compared to African-American, Latino, or American-Indian access. Many people who nominally have health insurance cannot afford to use it because of high deductibles and high copays, among other reasons. Insurance companies came up with deductibles and copays as tricks to increase their profits. If an individual has a $3,000 deductible per year, their insurance is useless unless they have a major hospitalization. Many who receive treatment that includes an ambulance ride or just one day in the hospital, end up burdened with overwhelming medical debt.

Since many people have no insurance, and many more others cannot afford to use their insurance because of copays or deductibles, many people do not seek treatment when they start having symptoms. Often, they have no idea what is causing the symptoms. Now, imagine the impact of having one person with an infectious disease who cannot afford to get tested or treated for that disease. How many in a community will be infected by that one untreated person and by all the others that one person infects? Now consider the number 30,000,000 and think about how many of those might have an infectious or otherwise dangerous illness. And let's include in that definition of "dangerous illnesses" any mental health condition that might cause someone to grab a kitchen knife and threaten to hurt themselves or a family member. What's the impact then?

The George Floyd protests in recent years have underscored, more starkly than ever, the urgent need to reevaluate the entire culture of police response. When a family member threatens to hurt themselves or others with a weapon, people have become understandably reluctant to call the police—mainly due to the many incidents of the police fatally shooting the individual who needs help (or even the individual who calls for help).

Even police departments admit that 20% of the calls they receive involve a mental health or substance use crisis.[100] From a public health point of view, it is important to consider the efforts that have been made to respond differently, and the lack of efforts in re-designing police training and promoting the mental health of police officers. In a study by the John Hopkins Bloomberg School of Public Health, 23% of shootings by police involved someone with a mental health issue—and of these shootings of mentally unhealthy persons, 67% were fatal.[101] A study by *Scientific American Magazine* found that Black males were twice as likely as white males to be killed by police.[102] Yale University found that despite the widespread use of police body cameras and increased media scrutiny of police shootings, the racial disparity in police shootings has remained unchanged.[103] *Mother Jones Magazine* reports that since George Floyd's murder by police, police killings have actually increased every year since 2020.[104] Poor mental health impacts not only victims of deadly police behavior, but it also impacts the police officers themselves.

A study by Walden University found that poor mental health continues to plague police departments, that more police officers die by suicide than by killings in the line of duty, and that the suicide rate for police officers is four times higher than that of firefighters. The same report said that less than 20% of police officers with a confirmed mental health issue sought help from professionals.

Apparently, the police culture continues to discourage mental health maintenance due to the stigma associated with it—a stigma ironically similar to the one that plagues physicians. Professionals who deal with life/death decisions are afraid to be seen as mentally unhealthy for fear that it will impact their careers. One way to interpret this is to suggest that seeking support for your own mental health carries more acknowledged career risk than harming yourself or members of the public. This is more than enough confirmation that there is a crisis in both the self-care culture and our public health practice when it comes to professionals upon whom our culture depends for protection.

There has been some progress in that at least 2,700 communities in the U.S. have developed Crisis Intervention Teams (CIT) that involve partnerships between mental health professionals and police officers. These partnerships help to reduce injuries to police officers and citizens, while also reducing costs. For example, NAMI points out that in Detroit the cost to keep a mentally unhealthy citizen in jail for one year is $31,000, compared to $10,000 per year to provide a similar citizen with community-based mental health support.[105]

Unfortunately, the 2,700 communities with CITs represent only about 15% of total police agencies in the U.S.[106] Even while CITs have helped reduce the killing of mentally unhealthy citizens, some cities have opted to remove police from CITs altogether.[107] Some have pointed out that there is little peer-reviewed evidence about the effectiveness of CITs.[108] More importantly, under the fluctuations of a dying capitalist system, there is no fundamental commitment to make the wellbeing of the citizenry the number one priority. Thus, as early as 2020 there were reports of cutbacks on CIT training.[109] In 2025, under the Trump administration, there have been major cuts to programs that support CIT.[110] Instead, the Trump administration has promoted police using more military equipment and artificial intelligence.[111] Overall, the Trump administration is reported to have cut spending on behavioral health and science related agencies by $29 billion.[112] Thus, future statistics about mental health and public health in the U.S. are bound to be worse. Even before the Trump administration, the U.S. ranked number 30 on a list of the countries with the best mental health. Government spending on mental health in the U.S. in 2023 was estimated at $2.40 per person, as compared to $10 per person in Sweden.[113]

Income inequality is correlated with lower levels of mental health. One professional journal estimated that "there are threefold differences in the proportion of the population suffering from mental illness between more or less equal countries."[114] Epidemiology professors Kate Pickett and Richard Wilkinson found that,

> Psychotic symptoms, such as delusions of grandeur, are more common in unequal countries, as is schizophrenia. Narcissism increases as income inequality increases... Those who live in more unequal places are more likely to spend money on expensive cars and to buy status goods; and are more likely to have high levels of personal debt because they try to prove that they are not second-class people by owning first-class things.[115]

The statistics on income inequality have become completely outrageous. According to the AFL-CIO, CEOs made 285 times more than workers in 2024. The CEO of Starbucks made 6,666 times as much as the company's median employee.[116] In 2023, the richest 1% in the world owned half of all the wealth, while the poorest half owned less than 1% of the wealth.[117]

Mental health is closely related to public health and all the policies that contribute to income and wealth inequality. This enmeshment suggests that a systematic change in economic system is the only solution. Any piecemeal reforms attempted while wealth inequality still exists are subject to reversal or neutralization. Wealthy people have a strong influence on who gets to run for office and who gets to stay in office. Government policies are subject to radical change depending on what politicians are in office. Politicians accepting money to support legislation favored by the wealthy is corruption, even if corruption has created laws that make that kind of corruption officially legal.

In the mental health field, corruption has even impacted how the diagnostic manual is written. Known as the *Diagnostic and Statistical Manual of Mental Disorders* (DSM) and published by the American Psychiatric Association, it's considered the "Bible" that provides clinicians guidelines to make a diagnosis. Insurance companies will not process a claim unless it includes one of their acceptable diagnoses drawn from the DSM. There have been only five editions of the DSM since 1952. By the time the fifth edition of the DSM was scheduled for release in 2013, many had grown frustrated with the extent of drug company influence over the professionals responsible for writing it. A well-respected journal published by the British Medical Association found that 60% of the panel and task force members for the DSM-5 had financial ties to industry. The same research disclosed that more than one third of panel members received compensation to serve as key opinion leaders, paid by the pharmaceutical industry to influence their peers. The British Medical Association labeled this arrangement as "an egregious financial conflict of interest."[118]

In the U.S., well before it is published, clinicians are made aware of any intended changes to the DSM. Thus, two weeks before the DSM-5 was to be published, the U.S. National Institute of Mental Health, the world's largest funding agency for mental health research, announced that it would no longer support the manual.[119] At minimum, this lack of faith in the manual is yet another indication that the entire mental health field needs a redesign. When this redesign can happen, it will be easier to consider mental health as public health. The entire point of taking a health approach instead of an illness approach is to promote the prevention of the disorders that the DSM is structured around. Private insurance companies support the DSM approach because they like to believe that a person's life needs to be significantly disordered by a problem before they qualify to use the mental health benefits they pay for.

One very prominent psychiatrist, Irvin Yalom, indicated that, except for certain specific psychotic disorders such as schizophrenia, "I personally avoid diagnosis entirely... Diagnosis is a negative form. It plays no role in the treatment I am providing..."[120] Fundamentally the present system is bankrupt, if only because we are using a diagnostic manual written primarily by people who are bribed by drug companies and supported by private insurance companies who are only interested in limiting care. We can do much better.

CHAPTER 6

GUIDELINES FOR GOOD MENTAL HEALTH

BERNARD NICOLAS

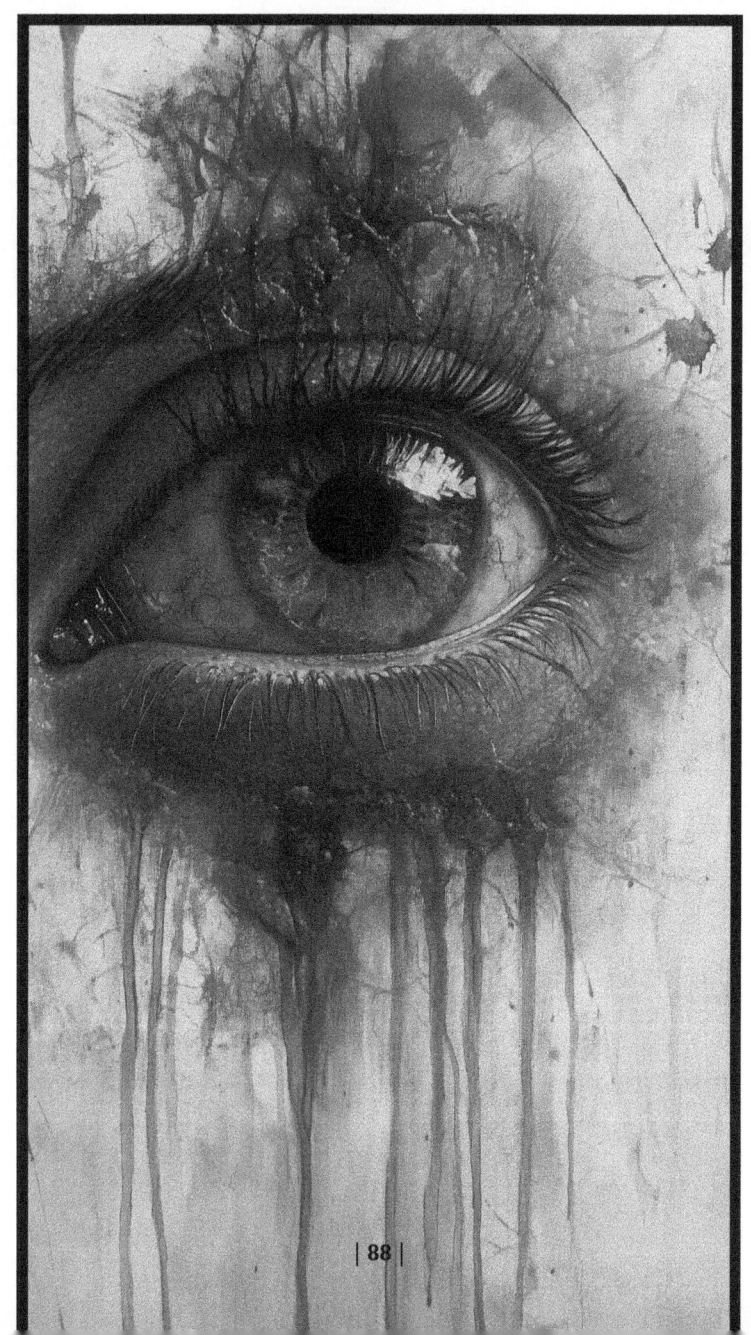

.....I KNOW KA-RAZY.... REJECTING THE CAPITALIST ROAD TO TWISTED MENTAL HEALTH

> **W**hat if we had commonly accepted indicators of what good mental health looks like, say something equivalent to the indicators we have for physical health?

If we don't know what we want or what it takes to get to what we want, then it is easier for sophisticated but corrupt politicians to sell us something that sounds good but is ultimately more of the same or worse. To illustrate, it's perhaps instructive to examine how the big "mangled care" companies managed to sell many of us on something called "Medicare Advantage."

For many decades, health care consumers as well as providers have wanted a universal single payer health care system. Such a system has sometimes been called "Medicare for All." When democratic socialist Bernie Sanders was running for president, there seemed to be some momentum toward consideration of Medicare for All. Yet this momentum did not seem to worry the big, mangled care companies. That is no doubt because they already had a counter strategy in place.

The concept of Medicare for All is to expand the federally run and administered Medicare system that pays providers to deliver health care needed by the population without restrictions, such as the current age-based eligibility. So-called Medicare Advantage is the opposite of Medicare for All in that it allows the mangled care companies to collect per member fees from our federal government and then restrict benefits delivered to the members in order to increase their profits. The door was open to mangled care companies when Congress passed laws in 1997 and 2003 that were presumably intended to improve the delivery of benefits that had previously not been a part of Medicare, such as prescription drug coverage.[121] The big for-profit insurance companies were so successful in selling Medicare Advantage that by 2024, 55% of all Medicare enrollees were under a Medicare Advantage plan. The profits of these companies also increased 287% between 2012 and 2024. Gradually, information began to emerge that some might consider scandalous. The mangled care companies were denying coverage for various health care services (even using AI to issue blanket denials) or were leaving members responsible for paying out-of-network fees for services from a provider that the member never realized was out of network.

With traditional Medicare, there is no such thing as in-network or out of network. There is also no pre-authorization requirement. A given provider either accepts Medicare or does not, and a procedure is either covered by Medicare or it is not. There is no uncertainly about getting pre-approval for health care treatment.

.....I KNOW KA-RAZY.... REJECTING THE CAPITALIST ROAD TO TWISTED MENTAL HEALTH

Medicare Advantage helped the seven biggest for-profit insurance companies increase their profits by $71.3 billion in 2024, while their CEOs took home a total of $146.1 million in compensation.[122] Meanwhile, in spite of news coverage regarding how mangled care is effectively stealing our tax dollars—albeit legally—Medicare Advantage continues to dominate the lives of individuals eligible for Medicare.

In summary, what has happened with Medicare Advantage is an example of how for-profit companies collaborate with corrupt politicians to provide the public with less health care. Thus, as we discuss the need for good mental health care, it is important to keep in mind that we are not likely to receive that good care from a dying capitalist system. Nevertheless, we need to know what good mental health care does or does not look like.

Even though some of our family members or neighbors may display clear signs of poor mental health, most of us do not feel qualified or confident enough to make a recommendation that an individual seek assistance. But what if we had commonly accepted indicators of what good mental health looks like, say something equivalent to the indicators we have for physical health?

According to Mind Help, good mental health is "about feeling connected, balanced, and capable—not just surviving, but actually living a fulfilling, happy, and complete life."[123] They suggest the following nine bullet points as characteristics of good mental health:

- Able to experience, express, and regulate a range of emotions
- Better able to deal with and recover from challenging situations
- Dealing with uncertainty and change in a healthy way
- Working towards achieving goals and realizing true potential
- Building and maintaining meaningful, healthy relationships
- Being aware of personal emotions and mood fluctuations
- Knowing how to set healthy personal boundaries
- Practicing self-love and self-care
- Having the ability to contribute to the community and feel a sense of belonging with others

There are various versions of the above indicators, and they are easy to find on the internet. So, the bigger question is not what should be the commonly accepted indicators, but why is a sense of mental health not as commonly accepted as indicators of good physical health? Part of the answer has to do with strong elements that are typical of an advanced stage of capitalism. These elements are huge investments in advertising intended to sell drugs and an accounting system that does not consider social costs or benefits. So, every day—if not every hour—we hear how the stock market is doing, but how

.....I KNOW KA-RAZY.... REJECTING THE CAPITALIST ROAD TO TWISTED MENTAL HEALTH

often do we hear that people are reporting feeling healthier or happier?

There are some major areas to consider relative to good mental health care. These are, prevention, access and empowerment.

If we start with **empowerment**, we soon realize that it is the key to ultimately accessing better health care and preventing a decline in our mental health. Empowerment runs counter to the culture that traditional capitalist health care has created. Even the use of the word patient reveals the preferred relationship that capitalist health care would like to have between us as people needing care and the big companies and authority figures (doctors) who provide the care. Patient comes from the Latin patior "meaning to suffer or bear whatever suffering is necessary and tolerating patiently the interventions of the outside expert."[124] The word doctor has its origins as a reference to a small group of theologians who "had approval from the Church to speak on religious matters."[125] No wonder the word continues to carry an implication of unquestionable authority even as it is used in health care. Just as most followers of a particular religion are not expected to question those who are approved to interpret the requirements of this religion, so too, patients are not expected to question the dictates of doctors. As the level of education in the general population has risen, so too has the audacity of people to question doctors and to realize that each of us has to be responsible for our wellbeing instead of expecting some authority figure who hardly knows us to be responsible for how we feel internally.

Once we are empowered, then we have the motivation and the energy to seek **access**. Finding the right health care often takes a lot of effort. We need to be able to understand what a particular provider's specialty is, whether that provider has any complaints or licensing restrictions, whether the provider accepts our insurance, whether the provider can see us in person (instead of telehealth), and whether the provider is likely to take the necessary time to get to know the history of our situation before whipping out the prescription form.

When we are empowered psychologically and we have some access to good health care information and treatment, then we can take steps to reduce the risk of a decline in our mental health.

But how can more people gain **access** to good health care under capitalism? It makes sense to continue to push for a universal single-payer health care system. Gallup poll results from 2023 indicate 57% of those polled believe the government should make sure everyone has health care coverage.[126] Not all of these responders believe health care should be provided through a Medicare-for-All type of system, though. The same poll shows 88% of Democrats believe the government should make sure all have coverage. Yet Hillary Clinton, as a Democratic candidate for president, infamously declared in

.....I KNOW KA-RAZY.... REJECTING THE CAPITALIST ROAD TO TWISTED MENTAL HEALTH

a debate with Bernie Sanders, "it will never, ever happen."[127] The myth of majority rule in the U.S. has been thoroughly debunked. A study done by political scientists Martin Gillens and Benjamin Page points out,

> In the United States, our findings indicate, the majority does *not* rule—at least not in the causal sense of actually determining policy outcomes. When a majority of citizens disagree with economic elites or with organized interests, they generally lose.[128]

So, we are not likely to get quality health care by supporting the Democratic Party or by simply voting for candidates who claim to support it. As Scott Tucker and Larry Gross pointed out,

> A successful campaign for the passage of a single-payer bill will require many tactics employed by many players. It will require a fully visible campaign that counters the attempts by politicians and their allies to divert, delay, and distort the analysis and directed anger: homework and hell raising. But, it can be done, because in the end, we are many and they are few.[129]

Another reason to push for universal single-payer health care is that if we can win with this very popular and fundamental issue, we will be well on our way to defeating capitalism. The major corporations that dominate health care, along with their political allies, are relying on their size and influence to prevent the majority from getting what we desperately need and want. This strategy is what sustains capitalism in every other industry. If we can defeat it in health care, we can do it in other areas of our economic life. Capitalism has failed to deliver quality health care for all—or even for the majority—and what's more the system has demonstrated repeatedly that profit for those in charge will always be the priority over quality of care.

.....I KNOW KA-RAZY.... REJECTING THE CAPITALIST ROAD TO TWISTED MENTAL HEALTH

While we struggle for quality health care, we still need to practice **prevention**. In the context of mental health, prevention means being aware that we need help to prevent a normal emotional reaction from turning into a deep-seated psychological issue. One way to do this is to think of emotional wounds in the same way we think of physical wounds. There are certain events and situations that happen in life that naturally cause a strong emotional response on our part. Life-threatening trauma, the death of a loved one, a deep betrayal, or severe abuse can easily be considered at least as serious psychologically as compound fractures in one or both legs would be physically. Just as a physical wound can lead to other complications, such as infection or damaging another part of the body while compensating for the broken limb, so can emotional wounds become more complicated. For example, experiencing betrayal as an adult can easily connect with a fear of abandonment in childhood that one might have thought had been dealt with and successfully suppressed.

The most important point, of course, is that you would never think of avoiding treatment for one or more compound fractures. You would also not think of treating a compound fracture yourself using band-aids, rubbing alcohol, and a needle and thread. If we begin to treat emotional wounds with the same urgency we apply to physical wounds, we can recognize that we need professional help. With that recognition, we can then go after the care we need. But without that recognition, we will let the wound get infected and we will hobble along until it kills us.

THE CAPITALIST ROAD: ARTIFICIAL SUGAR

BERNARD NICOLAS

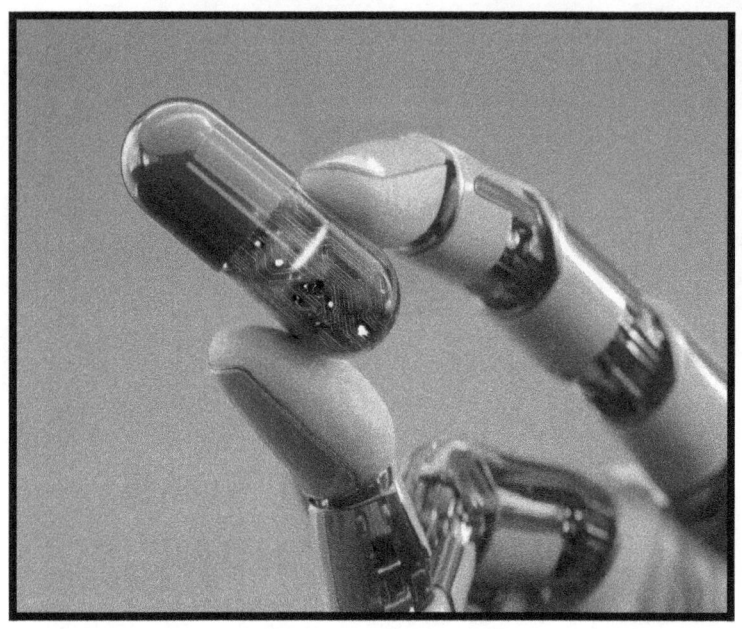

> The company that first marketed and sold heroin was Bayer AG (yes, the same outfit that still sells baby aspirin).

In the realm of capitalist thinking, any solution that involves fewer or preferably no humans is bound to be less costly and more predictable—at least until the horrible long-term side effects are revealed. Then it's a scandal and the capitalists come up with the next miracle solution. Evidence of this kind of thinking can be found in the development of artificial sugar.

.....I KNOW KA-RAZY.... REJECTING THE CAPITALIST ROAD TO TWISTED MENTAL HEALTH

The production of natural sugar played a major role in world history. Because sugar needed a warmer climate and because harvesting sugarcane and turning it into sugar required a lot of difficult labor, the demand for sugar in Europe was a tremendous incentive for African slavery and colonialism.[130] In the late 1800s a researcher accidentally discovered saccharin while looking for uses for biproducts of coal tar.[131] He had forgotten to wash his hands after lunch and licked his fingers. They tasted sweet. He ultimately discovered saccharin as he tried to figure out which of the coal tar biproducts produced the sweet taste.

Saccharin was used for many decades until it was found to be toxic. A similar pattern followed with the next three miracle sweeteners, cyclamate (aka Sweet'N Low), aspartame, and sucralose. We are currently in the pre-scandal phase of using xylitol. From the capitalist point of view, using a chemical that can be made in a lab, stored for long periods of time, and that provides a sweeter taste by volume compared to regular sugar is the only way to go. There is some talk today of trying to return to regular sugar, but this effort is not likely to be supported by the big capitalists.

When the capitalists apply their twisted thinking to the field of human mental health, they go through the same kinds of cycles as they did with artificial sugar.

Although it happened a long time ago, reexamining how the drug industry first marketed heroin can also in-form our current discourse. The company that first marketed and sold heroin was Bayer AG (yes, the same outfit that still sells baby aspirin). In the late nineteenth century, Bayer was a manufacturer of synthetic dyes made from coal tar, the same substance that the developer of saccharin was working with. In the summer of 1897, a Bayer employee found a way to transform the opiate morphine into a substance that was soon marketed as being more powerful and far less addictive than morphine. The brand name was "heroin" (meaning heroic in German). This medicine was so widely sold that one could order it from the Sears & Roebuck catalog. For $1.50 you could get a kit containing two vials of heroin, two syringes, two needles, and a handy carrying case.[132] Although a few doctors warned that this substance could be addictive, it was successfully sold for two decades as good medicine for pneumonia and a safe substitute for people who were dependent on morphine. Interestingly, about 100 years after the successful marketing of heroin, Purdue Pharma used a similar strategy to market oxycontin as a stronger and far less addictive pain reliever.[133] As with heroin, oxycontin was widely and successfully sold for a couple of decades, even though 806,000 people died from opioid overdoses between 1999 and 2023.[134] Oxy is still being prescribed and sold as of 2025, and the history of its marketing is an excellent example of how the capitalist drug industry has been able to market dangerous drugs to doctors and the public with relatively little interference from the Federal Drug Administration, the Drug Enforcement Administration, and other such agencies that are supposed to protect us.

Another outrageous capitalist notion is the alleged need to allow a legal monopoly to drug developers by issuing them patents. The big drug companies claim they need this "monopoly" to compensate for the cost of developing new drugs. In reality, taxpayers provide a large chunk of the cost of medical research. As of 2016, the National Institutes of Health was providing $30 billion annually for medical research.[135] During the COVID-19 pandemic, as of 2021, 98.12% of the funds spent to develop the vaccines came from taxpayers.[136] Yet 100% of the profits from these vaccines went to the capitalist companies selling them. These facts illustrate that there is no need to issue patents for drugs and that medicines should be treated as a public good.

Another trend found on the capitalist road is the medicating of children. Prescriptions of psychotropic drugs for young children doubled between 1995 and 2001.[137] One major contributing factor to this "drugging" of children comes from over diagnosing ADHD (Attention Deficit Hyperactivity Disorder). As pointed out by Dr. Suzanne O'Sullivan, an expert on neurological issues, "If you take a person with very severe ADHD and you do a brain scan for abnormalities, you will not find any abnormalities."[138] This means the criteria for diagnosing ADHD is essentially not reliable. As Dr. O'Sullivan also points out, the original intention for diagnosing ADHD or autism was to help people who have a great deal of trouble functioning. Vague diagnosing criteria has permitted the labeling of high-functioning individuals with ADHD or autism. One study found that children born within a few days of kindergarten or school cut-off dates are more likely to be diagnosed with ADHD. The study found that children born on one side of the cut-off date can be twice as likely to end up on stimulant prescriptions than children born a few days later but after the cut-off date.[139] The DSM criteria for ADHD has become more and more loose, and prescriptions for the stimulant drug Adderall (commonly prescribed for ADHD) have increased astronomically. From 2012 to 2023 dispensing of stimulants in the U.S. increased by 60%.[140] A significant percentage of people who use Adderall with or without a prescription do so because they feel it helps them function better in school. Some professionals suggest that if stimulant drugs help a person function better, it must be because they suffer from a disorder. But again, as Dr. O'Sullivan points out, if one gives testosterone injections to an athlete and she performs better, this does not mean that she had a testosterone deficiency.

There are other indicators for the over-prescription of drugs to children. One investigation found that 25% of children in foster care were being prescribed antipsychotic meds, not for mental illness but for behavior control.[141] This manner of prescribing drugs can easily be

.....I KNOW KA-RAZY.... REJECTING THE CAPITALIST ROAD TO TWISTED MENTAL HEALTH

considered child abuse, particularly because many psych meds have never been tested for their impact on children. One professor of psychology found that teens were being improperly prescribed antidepressants just for being sad. In some cases, the antidepressant drug ended up causing the child to complete suicide.[142] It is primarily because the drug business is so profitable that children are being overprescribed. One study found that 20% of children in the U.S. were on psychotropics.[143] Another contributing factor to the overuse of medication in capitalist medicine is that behavioral interventions are often overlooked or avoided because they cannot be monitored as efficiently as having a provider prescribe a drug and say, "Come back in three months." Particularly in children, there are multiple factors that can affect their behavior. Labeling a particular set of behaviors as a disease is a cynical way to make money, and it shows little concern for the long-term impact of medications on children.

Under capitalism, the costly part of good mental health is the part that involves the support of fellow human beings and creating healthy work and relaxation environments. Those settings to a capitalist are the equivalent of growing brown sugar in Cuba or Brazil and going through the costly transformations necessary to serve it as a uniformly bright and white powder in New York City or Paris. Capitalism would much rather treat mental health issues with drugs and AI bots because that is far more profitable and predictable. Even predictability has a different meaning in the capitalist context. It means that if profits with a certain drug are good in one year, we can make predictions about what the profit will be in the following year. Factors such as scandals caused by side effects are not factored into the capitalist predictability formula because they are, of course, too unpredictable.

Capitalism has already developed robot therapists. They will likely use one human licensed therapist to "monitor" 12 or more robot therapists. Then they will gradually reduce the human supervision as they collect "evidence-based" rationalizations. The capitalist answer to the mental health crisis is more chemistry and more technology. The fundamental difference between a capitalist approach and a socialist approach is about how humans are valued. Obviously, capitalists value capital more and socialists prioritize the value of human cooperation.

It cannot be a coincidence that, at the time of this writing, the U.S. is experiencing what some experts describe as "psychopathocracy." Professor Juan Cole defines psychopathocracy as "the rule of persons who lack a basic ability to empathize with others, to feel their pain, or to feel guilty about harming them."[144] Professor Steve Taylor points out that "pathological leaders always attract others with mental disorders... individuals who are moral, empathetic and fair-minded gradually fall away... pathocracies tend to become entrenched and extreme."[145] Dr. Taylor also points out that "pathocracies emerge only when citizens fail to take sufficient measures to protect themselves from maniacal leaders... all potential leaders should be rigorously assessed by mental health professionals for empathy, narcissism, selfishness, and psychopathy."

But how can a population that has not adopted a culture of mental health for everyone demand assessments of its leaders? Author Oliver James suggests that capitalism and bad mental health go together: "high levels of mental illness are essential to selfish capitalism, because needy, miserable people make greedy consumers and can be more easily suckered into perfectionist, competitive workaholism."[146]

A large study done in 2024 indicated that a population experiencing sadness, anger, or depression is more likely to vote for what the authors referred to as populist candidates, which could be either right-wing nationalists or left-wing socialists.[147] A study of Trump voters done in 2017 found that five phenomena—authoritarianism, social dominance, prejudice, lack of intergroup contact, and relative deprivation—"make people vulnerable to an intense sense of threat. Authoritarian leaders have long understood that they can attract followers by enhancing the perception of dangerous threats to the society and offering simple solutions."[148] Thus, we have a vicious cycle where lack of mental health makes possible the election of authoritarian leaders who exploit and promote that lack of mental health.

An increasing percentage of the population of the U.S. is rejecting the capitalist road. Some 70% of respondents in a recent survey said that the economic system is "rigged in favor of corporations and the wealthy" and needs to be replaced.[149] The same survey found that the majority of likely voters under 45 years old support socialism, with 83% of respondents also indicating that mental health should be a part of the public safety budget. The battle to transform the capitalist road completely will not be easy. But it helps that the majority of people are in favor of getting rid of capitalism.

DARE TO DREAM

BERNARD NICOLAS

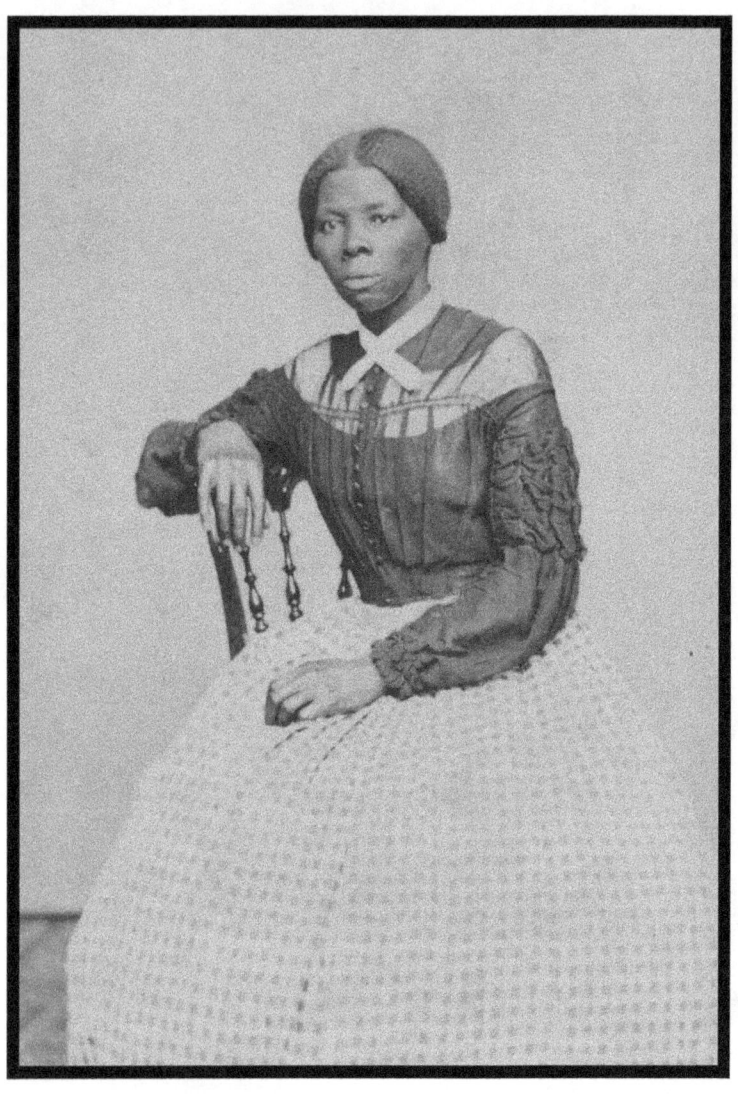

.....I KNOW KA-RAZY.... REJECTING THE CAPITALIST ROAD TO TWISTED MENTAL HEALTH

> The theory of how capitalism is supposed to work is even more abstract than theories about how socialism can work.

A common tool used in clinical psychology is visualization. The idea is to visualize the change you want so clearly and consistently that it strengthens your belief that it's achievable. At this point in countries plagued by dying capitalism, there are only two main options, either a socialist future or a post-apocalyptic one like we have been shown in many movies. It is perhaps no coincidence that the capitalist film industries would rather have us visualize a scary future of disaster and/or fascism, rather than a peaceful one where socialism allows the kind of love and collaboration that makes amazing human advancement possible. Occasionally, the capitalist film industries create a product that presents a point of view that is critical of capitalism. One such film was released in 1975 under the title *Rollerball* and is summarized by one reviewer as follows:

BERNARD NICOLAS

In the world of *Rollerball*, the titular sport serves as both a brutal entertainment spectacle and a tool for the ruling corporations to suppress dissent and unify the populace under a veneer of camaraderie. Jonathan E., an exceptional athlete, initially revels in the admiration that his prowess brings. However, as he discovers the sinister motivations of the corporate entities that control his life, his position of power becomes increasingly precarious. The executives, determined to maintain their monopoly, target him as a symbol of individuality that threatens their absolute dominance over society. As the plot unfolds, Jonathan begins to fight against the corporate machinations that threaten his identity and the very essence of the sport he loves... The film culminates in a harrowing climax, where the true cost of resistance is laid bare amid the chaos of the Rollerball arena, revealing not only the brutality of the sport but also the fragility of personal freedom in the face of an indifferent corporate machine.[150]

.....I KNOW KA-RAZY.... REJECTING THE CAPITALIST ROAD TO TWISTED MENTAL HEALTH

Rollerball was exceptional in that it shows a capitalist future that is full of abundance, technology, and engaging distractions. At the same time, independent thinking is brutally suppressed. The film stared James Caan and was directed by prolific director Norman Jewison, yet it is not shown regularly on streaming channels—perhaps because it carries an uncomfortable truth. As the reviewer put it, "it is not simply an entertaining spectacle but a cautionary tale that is increasingly relevant today." It is difficult to watch *Rollerball* and not think about how big corporations who control our lives today want to keep us distracted while coming down hard on individuals who dare to put ideas forward that the corporations find counterproductive to their interests. (Think Colin Kaepernick and the NFL.)

Clinical psychology has shown that optimism tends to produce better real-world outcomes than pessimism. In other words, if a devastating earthquake were to occur and you and I were trapped under rubble, I might despair and wail that this is the end and we're all going to die, while you admit the situation is terrible, but suggest we try moving some debris to see if we can escape. Research shows that you, the optimist, are more likely to survive than I, the pessimist.[151] Thus, in the spirit of optimism, this writer declares that the U.S. will soon be on its way to a bright socialist future. The horror that we are seeing now under the Trump presidency represents part of the death spasms of a dying system. What then will this socialist future look like and how will mental health be promoted under such an economic system?

In order for a visualization to work it needs to be somewhat grounded in reality. If you are a short adult, you can visualize yourself as being six feet tall. The visualization may help you feel tall, but it is not likely to allow you to actually become tall. As we visualize socialism in a country like the U.S., it is helpful to look at some facts that already exist. How socialism would work is not just a utopian pipe dream. Economist Richard Wolff has done a lot of work on viewing socialism in terms of worker-owned workplaces. He points out that examples of this kind of workplace already exist:

> Worker co-ops have a long history and a wide presence in today's world. To take one leading example of the many thousands of worker co-ops across the world, the Corporacion Mondragon in the Basque region of Spain offers over half a century's experience as proof of the viability of this economic model. Mondragon started with six workers and now includes over 80,000. It is now one of Spain's 10 largest corporations.[152]

.....I KNOW KA-RAZY.... REJECTING THE CAPITALIST ROAD TO TWISTED MENTAL HEALTH

While we already have some concrete examples of how new socialist workplaces could function, it is not necessary that we figure out every detail of how a socialist system would work in the future. As Wolff points out,

> A new economy based on worker co-ops will have to find its own democratic way to structure relationships among co-ops and society as a whole. Such an economy will need to work out, for instance, the best proportion of planned versus market distributions, and private versus public workplace ownership, as well as determine the specific structure of laws and regulations.[153]

This means that under a new socialism, free enterprise can still exist, and entrepreneurs will be able to own businesses. The only restriction will be to prevent the legal exploitation of workers on a large scale.

Some people may not know that there are large employers in the U.S. today that are employee owned. One such example is Publix Supermarkets. Their 255,000 employees own the largest block of shares, while the founder's family owns the next largest block, and the employee retirement plan owns the third largest block. The employees therefore have a chance to vote on corporate matters. It's only one example, but it demonstrates that it is possible to structure economic enterprises in ways that do not give private capital full control.[154]

Another interesting fact might help us better visualize a more equitable distribution of wealth: if all the wealth in the U.S. were distributed equally, each person (adult or child) would have an estimated $471,465. That would mean $942,930 per couple, or $1.89 million for a couple with two children.[155] This statistic is just a way of illustrating that there is already enough wealth in the country for every single resident to have a much better life.

Another area to consider is the rapid advancement of technology. We now have machines that can control other machines that can then make a lot of the products previously manufactured by human labor. According to a 2016 report, 39% of the U.S. workforce is likely to be replaced by automation. Another report by the Economic Policy Institute finds that between 2000 and 2017, the U.S. economy lost $2 trillion in wages unpaid due to automation.[156]

Capitalists see this technological progress as a battle between greater profits and unemployment. Socialists see these developments as the basis for a good standard of living with more leisure time.

Prior to capitalism, the development of tools tended to improve quality of life. Under capitalism, however, technology is often used to increase profits by reducing the workforce while demanding the same level of labor from fewer workers. Meanwhile, wealthier capitalists have used their higher incomes to drive up the cost of housing and other essentials, thereby making life even harder for working people.[157]

Economist Richard Wolff explains clearly how the use of technology would change if all major employers became co-ops run by the workers. Technology could be used to maintain the same level of output, while allowing workers to earn the same wages, but work less.[158] With significantly more leisure time, many workers could choose to be of service to their communities by taking children on field trips or spending time recording stories with the elderly about their memories (this reduces loneliness among the elderly while making them feel valued and producing a lot of audio/visual history).

Under capitalism, the culture of working to pay bills, using commodities to prop up our self-esteem, and using substances to escape our drudgery—all add up to poor mental health. Under a new and never-before-seen kind of socialism, holistic health care can be available to all, low-cost preventive mental health activities such as group exercise and meditation can be promoted, and peer support can characterize significant parts of our lives from dealing with grief to creating public art.

Some people may feel as if socialism is still an abstraction while capitalism is real. Such skeptics should keep in mind that the theory of how capitalism is supposed to work is even more abstract than theories about how socialism can work. In order for capitalism to really function as a free enterprise economy controlled by markets, there are certain assumptions that are necessary in the capitalist theory of micro-economics. Some of these assumptions are...

1. Buyers and sellers have free and complete access to information
2. Businesses can easily enter or leave markets at will without significant obstacles
3. There are many buyers and sellers in the market so that no single entity can influence pricing

Just these three assumptions clearly demonstrate what an abstract concept the theory of capitalist micro-economics represents.[159] Under capitalism, we certainly do not have free access to information. Subscriptions to information services such as Lexis Nexis for example run $1,878/month. Rich people who share stock tips at the country club golf course are not making the same information available to poor people waiting in line at the retail bank. In most industries under capitalism there are huge obstacles to entering or leaving a market. A bakery owner cannot decide on a whim to leave that business and get into car manufacturing. The bakery owner would not be able to get a loan to start a car factory, and the baker's knowledge about baking would not attract investors because that knowledge does not transfer to car manufacturing. Finally, most major industries under capitalism, such as airlines, weapons manufacturers, entertainment companies, or even health care are dominated by a handful of large corporations, each of which could easily influence prices.

The talk about free enterprise under capitalism is a con game. Interestingly, all con games require the mark to believe the picture the con artist is painting. Similarly with capitalism, we are led to believe that the $100 bill we hold in our hands has value beyond the cost of the paper it is printed on. In reality that $100 bill's value could drop down to 1 cent on any given day because there is no concrete substance backing its value. If people lose faith in banks and just half of the customers go in all at once and demand their money, the entire capitalist economy would collapse in a couple of weeks. That's because, for every dollar a bank holds in its vault, it is allowed to lend out $15—effectively creating a money supply that exists only on paper. As of March 15, 2020, the reserve requirement was dropped to 0% which means banks are not legally required to have any actual real cash to back up the loans they give out.[160] Under this kind of wild capitalism, banks are highly vulnerable to failure, which in turn makes the entire capitalist system susceptible to collapse.

For those who want and believe in socialism, the challenge is not trying to imagine the collapse of capitalism, because that part is really easy to imagine. The real challenge is believing and imagining widespread democracy at work, elected leaders who are not corrupt, and public policy that prioritizes good health and peace of mind for everyone.

Picture that and tell yourself it's possible. It takes daring and courage to allow yourself to pursue what seems like only a dream. It also takes courage to go against the establishment and challenge the status quo.

Leadership coach Jill Schulman points out that bravery is not something we are born with. It is a skill that we must practice. And when we practice it, we are actually training the part of our brain that controls planning and decision-making. As this bravery muscle gets stronger, it becomes easier to do the next scary thing. Schulman also explains that it helps to surround ourselves with other people who take on big goals and walk through fear. Thus, the mutual courage rubs off. Finally, Schulman recommends that we can train ourselves to see fear not as a sign of danger but as an opportunity for growth.[161]

CHAPTER 9

PSYCHOLOGY OF LIBERATION

BERNARD NICOLAS

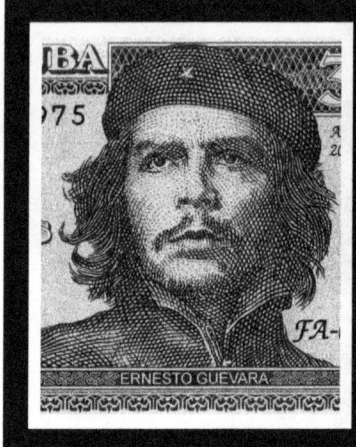 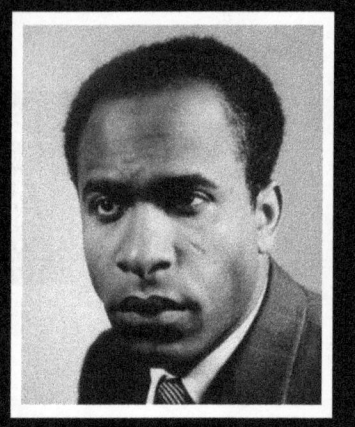

> ... we are each other's harvest:
> We are each other's
> business:
> We are each other's
> magnitude and bond.
> -Gwendolyn Brooks

The psychology of liberation involves at least one complex contradiction in that the mindset necessary to make radical change is not necessarily the mindset we will want once that radical change has been established. Although many people want to think that a revolution should be able to happen peacefully, such an outcome is highly unlikely. We are already seeing political violence such as beatings, car rammings, and assassinations—and the revolution has not even started. We also know that violent conflict is likely to be psychologically harmful. There is a quote attributed to highly decorated war hero David Hackworth that suggests that conflict is not at all about fighting fair: "If you find yourself in a fair fight, you didn't plan your mission properly."[162]

Many people today admire the warrior mindset and promote it as if it were a positive path to success. In reality, conflict causes ugly scenes, and ugly scenes often cause PTSD. Psychotherapist Edward Tick, author of *War and the Soul*, points out that "we deny that war changes its participants forever, promoting instead the belief that PTSD can be repaired and that vets and survivors can resume an ordinary civilian identity."[163] Tick believes that PTSD is not a psychological but a soul disorder that impacts a warrior's morality, spirituality, and even his/her sense of intimacy.[164] He later outlines how ancient cultures viewed the condition as a communal rather than an individual problem. He describes how Native American cultures such as the Papago people held a "sixteen-day purification ceremony for young warriors when they returned from their first experiences of taking life. During this ceremony they were tended only by old warriors, so that they had the benefit of their elder's experience to facilitate their transition back to civilian life."[165] The point is that pre-revolutionary conflict, as well as revolutionary conflict, is psychologically damaging. Preparations must be made in advance to help those who are traumatized by it to heal as much as possible.

One major driver of human motivation is identity, which is fueled by the need to belong. In the process of radical change, our sense of identity is challenged and often permanently altered. Any successful radical change will need to promote healing, partly through the development of healthier identities, such as the "New Man" discussed in more detail below.

Several important writers have commented on elements related to the psychology of liberation. Clearly a major psychological factor in the radical change process is that there comes a time when the current conditions cannot accommodate the many people with a passion for change. To paraphrase C.L.R. James "passion not spent but turned inward… torn, twisted, stretched to the limits of agony, injected with poisonous patent medicines" can lead to death or to liberation.[166] Frantz Fanon, a psychiatrist and avid promoter of the Algerian Revolution pointed out that,

.....I KNOW KA-RAZY.... REJECTING THE CAPITALIST ROAD TO TWISTED MENTAL HEALTH

> The fight carried out by a people for its liberation leads it, according to circumstances, either to refuse or else to explode the so-called truths which have been established in its consciousness by the colonial civil administration, by the military occupation, and by economic exploitation. Armed conflict alone can really drive out these falsehoods created in man which force into inferiority the most lively minds among us and which literally mutilate us.[167]

Fanon published *Wretched of the Earth* in 1963, but his work continues to be seminal in the present wherever there is a situation that calls for radical change. His mention of armed conflict suggests that carrying out such conflict can heal some parts of the oppressed psyche. But as discussed above, conflict can also cause new harm. In Algeria, Fanon urged his comrades not to imitate Europe but to,

> ... flee from this motionless movement where gradually dialectic is changing into the logic of equilibrium. Let us consider the question of mankind. Let us consider the question of cerebral reality and of the cerebral mass of all humanity, whose connections must be increased, whose channels must be diversified and whose messages must be re-humanized.[168]

Writing some 33 years later, psychiatrist Aaron Beck, the great theoretician of cognitive behavioral therapy, echoed Fanon as he praised Dr. Leslie Brothers who,

> ... demonstrated how our brains have evolved a specialized capacity for 'exchanging signals' with other brains. She suggests that even individual neurons respond to social events... The challenge of the next millennium will be to utilize these wellsprings to provide a more benevolent climate for the human race.[169]

.....I KNOW KA-RAZY.... REJECTING THE CAPITALIST ROAD TO TWISTED MENTAL HEALTH

Beck makes a strong argument that the opposite of "group narcissism" is "enlightened altruism." He also points out that one individual who risked his life to save a child claimed that if he had not acted, he would have "died inside."[170] Poet Gwendolyn Brooks, in a tribute to the activist Paul Robeson wrote,

> ... we are each other's harvest:
> We are each other's
> business:
> We are each other's
> magnitude and bond.[171]

All of these writers seem to agree that radical change can be motivated by altruism and by a love for and sense of connection with our fellow humans.

Human beings have a fundamental need to belong, to socially identify with a group of other humans. Groups in turn "influence behavior because they create a collective identity for all members. This collective identity is shaped by both in-group cohesion and out-group hostility."[172]

For the revolutions of the twentieth century, nationalism was a major identity anchor. Now in the twenty-first century, with capitalism having fully intertwined the world economy and with social media and other internet-based applications, people have different identity anchors that transcend national boundaries. The TikTok ban illustrates the international character of social media and the powerlessness of national governments. In January 2025, a genocidal war was going on in Gaza and TikTok was a very popular app used by young people all over the world. Some U.S. politicians were apparently upset that they could not control news clips seen by young citizens that were severely tarnishing Israel's image.[173] They then pretended that TikTok needed to be banned for fear that the Chinese might be stealing valuable data that would endanger the security of the U.S. Before the politicians could even complete their attack on TikTok, a large portion of TikTok users who dubbed themselves "TikTok refugees" shifted to a different app (also based in China) called RedNote.[174] Clearly, young social media users do not subscribe to the paranoid nationalist mentality of old.

One fundamental lesson gifted to us by the twentieth century revolutions is the notion of the "New Man" and the "New Woman." Argentine-born Cuban revolutionary Ernesto Che Guevara is one of the leaders who articulated the concept well. His point of view is described as follows:

.....I KNOW KA-RAZY.... REJECTING THE CAPITALIST ROAD TO TWISTED MENTAL HEALTH

> For Che, every revolutionary should strive to exemplify the new socialist man in their actions, through being honest, hardworking, incredibly studious, and willing to labor for the good of the collective society. This marks a radical transition away from the capitalist notion of growth centered on an individual's accumulation of capital and commodities, and towards a socialist notion of growth centered on human flourishing—towards a notion of the human being as the unique expression of the ensemble of relations they are embedded in as individuals dialectically interconnected to the social.[175]

In his own essay on revolutionary medicine, Guevara suggested that medical doctors will need to change both their thinking and their actions. He felt doctors must think of themselves partly as farmers and partly as politicians, and that,

> ... the first thing we will have to do is not go to the people to offer them wisdom. We must go, rather, to demonstrate that we are going to learn with the people, that together we are going to carry out that great and beautiful common experiment: the construction of a new Cuba.[176]

It is thanks to this kind of inspiration that Cuban health care is now considered much better than that of the U.S. And Cuban doctors have served many populations throughout the world free of charge.

The concept of transforming ourselves is closely related to the enlightened altruism that Beck wrote about and the "being each other's harvest" that Brooks included in her poem. Thus, our in-group cohesion can potentially be based on the love of our common humanity.

But what about our out-group hostility? How should we define the enemy? And must we hate that enemy in order to maintain our in-group cohesion?

During the Occupy Movement of the early twenty-first century, the notion of the "One Percent" emerged as the potential enemy. This concept is valuable if only because it reminds us that the enemy is numerically small—and that we, the 99%, are clearly the vast majority. The horrendous wealth inequality around the world helps to sub-

.....I KNOW KA-RAZY.... REJECTING THE CAPITALIST ROAD TO TWISTED MENTAL HEALTH

stantiate the notion that the coming revolution will be about the power of the 99% vs. the power of the 1%.

To maintain its power, the 1% clearly uses a lot of violence. There has never been a revolution that did not find the need to use violence to counter the enemy's often institutionalized violence. But violence cannot be a primary tactic for a revolution that is inspired by love. Creativity—one more powerful than anything AI can generate—is more likely to be our most successful tactic. To the extent that some of us will find ourselves being either survivors or perpetrators of violence, we will need to heal. Healing and maintaining good mental health is what the next chapter is about.

BERNARD NICOLAS

MAINTAINTING MENTAL HEALTH

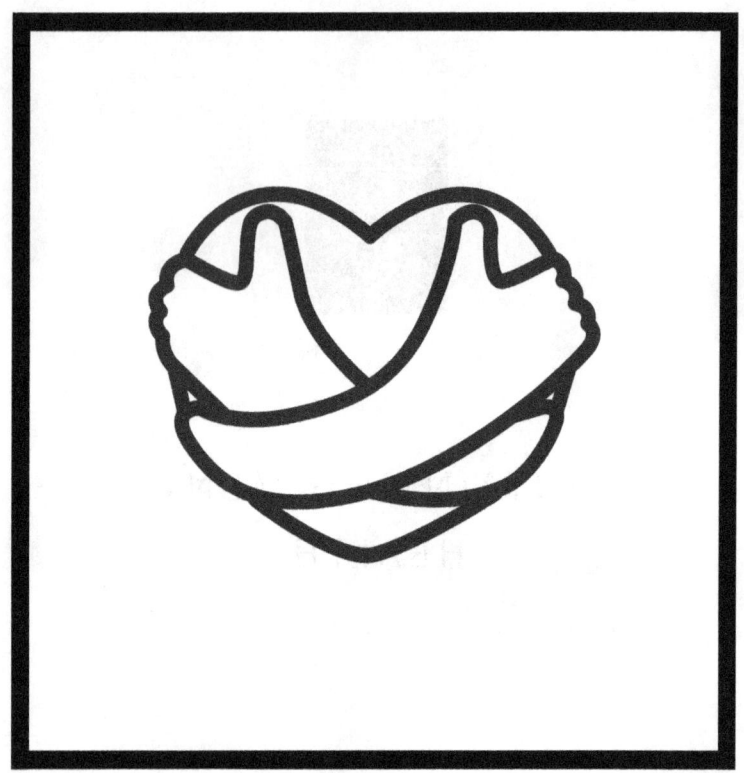

> One key element of mental health that will be important before, during, and after the revolution is self-care.

Many ancient cultures thrived for hundreds if not thousands of years before their societies were disrupted by European colonization. This is not an attempt to romanticize those strong cultures in Africa, Asia, and the areas that the Europeans would later arrogantly label as the Americas. Instead, the point is that maintaining mental health is not a new challenge that has never been addressed before. Ancient cultures nurtured a strong connection to nature; their fundamental thinking was community oriented, and their medicine was based on traditional healing systems. There were no copays, prior authorizations, or denials. Their self-care was rooted in spirituality, ceremony, and ritual.

Thus, one key element of mental health that will be important before, during, and after the revolution is self-care. Once we are mature enough to practice self-care, it becomes the most important thing we do.

Prioritizing self-care is a coping strategy.

No one else is responsible for our wellbeing. No one usually knows our bodies and our minds better than we are capable of knowing them. There are obvious forms of physical self-care such as hygiene, good nutrition, and proper rest. When it comes to mental self-care, the first step is to be motivated, to remind yourself that you are valuable to your community and that you have a responsibility to take care of your mind whether you feel like it or not. This is similar to the notion of eating even when we are not hungry or in the mood for it, such as when we are in deep grief. We eat anyway, because we know that our body needs fuel to survive.

There are many types of activities that can promote self-care, ranging from taking a relaxing bath, to a beauty treatment, meditation, prayer, exercise, making artwork or crafts, playing music, or doing volunteer work that gives you a sense of purpose and makes you feel good about being part of your community.

In our busy and stressful lives, there are many forces that can interfere with self-care. It is not possible to practice regular self-care unless you take a determined attitude to do it daily. Even if it is only for five minutes at the beginning of the day, it is helpful because, in those few minutes, you can remind yourself that self-care is important and that you need to make time to do more of it.

An element of mental health related to self-care is enforcing boundaries. Given the strain of our current troubled and unhealthy culture, people often feel entitled to disregard personal boundaries in pursuit of their own needs. If someone tries to prevent you from doing your self-care or pushes you to participate in some unhealthy behavior (even after you have told them "no" once), you have to step up your boundary enforcement efforts even at the risk of appearing rude. In the long run, it's better to risk upsetting a friend, family member, or acquaintance than to compromise your mental health. Each of us has to practice developing our own calm but assertive voice to enforce our boundaries.

Having and enforcing boundaries is another coping strategy.

.....I KNOW KA-RAZY.... REJECTING THE CAPITALIST ROAD TO TWISTED MENTAL HEALTH

Just as you enforce boundaries with others, it is important to manage your self-talk. Self-talk is your inner voice. It is a voice that has been influenced by a number of factors. It is sometimes positive, but most of the time it is negative or at least counterproductive. For many of us, our inner voice chatters so constantly that we are often not aware of it. It is like a subliminal background message. We may not be paying attention to it, but it affects us constantly.

Thus, the first thing to do is be aware of our self-talk, and the second thing is to realize we can talk back to it, reframe it, ignore it, or teach it how to be more positive. For example, your self-talk might tell you, "You could never do this, you are not ____ enough!" You now have the option to reframe this message as, "Yes, this is a huge undertaking, but maybe I can break it down into small chunks and deal with each chunk one at a time!"

Managing your self-talk is an important coping strategy.

Another important aspect of mental health is avoiding the use of substances—such as food, alcohol, prescription medication, or other drugs—to mask discomfort or pain. Sitting in discomfort or manageable pain can be healthy. It can often lead to writing a poem, composing a song, or capturing your feelings in a drawing or painting. Capitalist culture has tried very hard to convince us to buy products to make us feel good at all times. This attitude is unhealthy and creates the foundation for behavioral and substance addiction.

Abusing substances or denying addiction is an unhealthy coping strategy.

Seeking help from professionals or 12-step groups is a reliable way to stop using and to learn healthy coping strategies. Severe pain, such as that which follows a major surgery, is a different matter. Severe pain should be managed with advice and/or prescriptions from a competent professional.

Like all ancient cultures did, nurturing our spirituality is vital. Broadly defined, spirituality is involved in any thought or activity that involves a concern beyond our individual existence. Being aware that I am part of a family, a neighborhood, a human race, visiting a museum, or being intimate with another person—these are all forms of spirituality. Intellectual notions of being atheist, agnostic, or religious are a different matter. Spirituality can be practiced individually or with a group, but it is always connected to our species-being. Species-being is a Marxist term that basically means that one is aware that "nature is his body, with which he must remain in continuous interchange if he is not to die." Marx further states that a conscious being is "one that treats the species as its own essential being, or that treats itself as a species being."[177] In this context then, to fail to practice spirituality is a way of shortchanging your existence as a human.

Nurturing your spirituality is another healthy coping strategy.

To maintain your physical and mental health, it is also important to use the flawed health care system, particularly for the things that it does best, namely its diagnostic tools. If you think you have a bone fracture, you need to demand an x-ray. If you think you have a brain tumor, you can demand an MRI. Or, if you think you have cancer, you need a biopsy. The main points here are that...

1. it's important to detect problems early with the right diagnostic tools
2. regardless of your insurance coverage or lack thereof, you are entitled to the best health care available, and you have to fight to get it.

There are people who have top-notch private insurance who die unnecessarily simply because they accept a doctor telling them they don't need this or that test.

Having regular health check-ups is another healthy coping strategy.

As corrupt as the capitalist health care system has been, it does save lives. Similarly, the pharmaceutical industries are also corrupt, but there are some health conditions that currently can only be managed with medication. Examples are Type 1 diabetes which requires insulin injections, or severe psychotic symptoms that only antipsychotic drugs can manage in the short run.

If you have a condition that can only be managed with medication, it is important to take that medication as prescribed and avoid completely running out of it.

Following through on treatment recommendations is another healthy coping strategy.

Being alone and enjoying your own company is called solitude. Solitude can be an opportunity to relax or practice self-care. Avoiding other people for unhealthy reasons is called isolation. According to the CDC, social isolation can increase the risk of having heart disease and stroke, suicidal depression, dementia, or early death.[178] Obviously, isolation is something to avoid. In our current culture, it often takes a lot of effort to avoid isolation. People are distrustful of others, and there are plenty of distractions to provide a false sense of being engaged. Among these distractions are social media, or the soon to be popular virtual reality. None of these is an adequate substitute for face-to-face human interaction.

Avoiding isolation is a healthy coping strategy.

Interacting with other humans is bound to occasionally result in anger. Anger is often temporary, but resentments can last a long time. Anger is a normal human emotion that Carlos Todd, PhD, LCMHC differentiates from resentment as follows:

.....I KNOW KA-RAZY.... REJECTING THE CAPITALIST ROAD TO TWISTED MENTAL HEALTH

> Anger... is typically a response to a perceived threat, frustration, or injustice. On the other hand, resentment goes beyond the immediate reaction of anger. It involves harboring long-lasting bitterness... and deep-seated negativity toward another person, situation, or event.[179]

Resentment, as some describe it, is like taking poison in order to punish another person. It is important to process and release resentments. This can be done by managing self-talk or doing a fourth-step (typically a deep, honest examination of your past actions, thoughts, and behaviors as part of a 12-step recovery process) or talk-therapy or praying—or all of the above. But emotions like anger can be channeled in a positive direction rather than being suppressed. If you find yourself angry at some aspect of the failing capitalist system, it is important for you to own your anger and remind yourself that you have a choice on how you choose to react to injustice. If you let the system or anybody else be responsible for your anger, then you cannot manage it because it is beyond your control. However, if you own your anger, you can choose to channel it into positive action to change the system that provoked it.

Nurturing emotional maturity is another healthy coping strategy.

Author Tricia Hersey encourages us to view rest not as a luxury to indulge in when convenient, but as an intentional and affirming practice,

> Rest is a spiritual practice.
> Rest is a justice practice...
> Rest is an anti-capitalist practice.
> Rest is a freedom-seeking practice.[180]

Hersey goes on to write,

> ...Burnout is a scam and its language was created by agents of grind culture, guided by corporations tricking you into believing it's a normal and regular part of any working person's career. We speak the word 'burnout' so much when it should be named correctly instead. There is no 'burnout.' There is worker exploitation, abuse from capitalism, and trauma stored in our bodies from a lifetime of overworking.[181]

.....I KNOW KA-RAZY.... REJECTING THE CAPITALIST ROAD TO TWISTED MENTAL HEALTH

The main point is that adequate rest is fundamental to all mental health concerns. We must avoid the attitude that pushing ourselves to function on very little sleep is somehow heroic. It is actually foolish and self-destructive. There are times when we cannot avoid pushing ourselves by reducing rest time. But when these things happen, it is important to recover and catch up on rest. Most revolutionary movements do not happen under ideal conditions. Often leaders at all levels are pushed to do more and more, leading to burnout. As much as possible, this scenario needs to be avoided by using collective leadership. Collective leadership also prevents the enemy from harassing particular leaders and driving them toward a decline in mental health.

Making sure you get good quality rest is a healthy coping strategy.

One final element of mental health can appear to be contradictory because it is about accepting what you cannot change, yet having the courage to change the things you can. This apparent contradiction is well captured by the spirit of *The Serenity Prayer*. The practice of acceptance is mentioned here because it is an effective way to reduce anxiety and stress.

Particularly for people who are trying to bring about the kind of radical change most people dare not think about, it is important to know when to let a particular campaign go and when to take up one that others may think is foolish. Spirituality can be a guideline in making these choices. This is because spirituality helps to bring calm reflection, and it is easier to consider the greater good or the most strategic objective when one is calm and not driven by ego or reactivity.

Balancing acceptance with the courage to make changes is yet another healthy coping strategy.

Author bell hooks, in her book *all about love*, writes, "it takes courage to befriend death. We find that courage in life through loving."[182] To love myself and to love my fellow humans means making the best of each day, enjoying life, and being of service to my various communities. If I can do that, I have absolutely no reason to fear death. The fear of death can only prevent me from enjoying the day that I am in. What I have feared far more than death is having a meaningless and purposeless life.

Making each day of my life as meaningful as possible is a healthy coping strategy.

ABOUT THE AUTHOR

Bernard Nicolas's life trajectory has taken him from being a Catholic altar boy to a Black militant student organizer, and from a self-centered alcoholic to a spiritually-oriented psychotherapist. He has also been a filmmaker, parent, novelist, and photographer.

His family emigrated from Haiti when he was 11 years old.

He holds a B.A and M.F.A. from the University of California Los Angeles, and an M.A. in Clinical Psychology from Antioch University Los Angeles. He has been a Licensed Marriage and Family Therapist for more than 20 years.

As a child, Bernard often heard the Vodun drums coming from the mountains of Haiti and connecting him to Africa and the seminal Haitian Revolution. Today, he still hears those drums in his mind—a constant and rhythmic reminder that a better world is coming.

ACKNOWLEDGMENTS

I first want to acknowledge my higher power and the ancestral spirits that allowed me to salvage my own mental health. I am also grateful to the many individuals who showed me how—and encouraged me—to think critically about daring to challenge the status quo.

At Antioch University Los Angeles, I especially appreciated the insights and support of instructors such as Dr. Sylvie Taylor, who inspired me to specialize in community psychology, and Dr. Viktor Sigalov who introduced me for the first time to the real history of health care and psychopharmacology in the U.S.

I continue to benefit from the love and support of my fellowship mates in my 12-step program, where we have many useful slogans. One of these is "uncover, discover, and discard."

I pray that this little book of mine will help move us closer to discarding the failed capitalist health care system. I am grateful to all the "ka-razies" who allowed me to see how their minds worked—among them are beloved family members, cherished friends, and a few ever-annoying acquaintances.

PHOTO CREDITS

Chapter 1: Baby - Adobe stock

Chapter 2: Suicidal MD - Adobe stock

Chapter 3: Sisters hugging - Eye for Ebony on Unsplash

Chapter 3: Egyptian sarcophagus - B. Nicolas

Chapter 4: Cop - Adobe stock

Chapter 5: Wounded Eye - Adobe stock

Chapter 6: Robot with pill - Adobe stock

Chapter 7: Harriet Tubman - Library of Congress - Benjamin F. Powelson

Chapter 8: Che Guevarra - Adobe stock

Chapter 9: Frantz Fanon - Public Domain

Chapter 10: Self-care graphic - Adobe stock

Front Cover:

Timothy McVeigh - Public Domain – FBI mug shot

Shamsud Din-Jabbar - Licensed from FBI/ZumaPress/Alamy Photos

Seung-Hui Cho - Licensed from Virginia State Police/Alamy Photos

Christopher Dorner - Licensed from Alamy Photos

Donald Trump - Library of Congress Public Domain photo

Back Cover:

Author photo - M Fort Photo

END NOTES

1. African proverb, "He who has health has hope, and he who has hope has everything," quoted in *African Sayings About Health*, Sayings Collection, accessed November 2025, https://sayings.mingyanjiaju.org/african-sayings-about-health.

Introduction

2. Jesus Mesa, "As Gold Hits New Record, Some See Warning Signs of Civilizational Collapse," *Newsweek*, accessed October 2025, https://www.newsweek.com/why-gold-prices-are-soaring-10849599.
3. Richard D. Wolff, *Understanding Socialism*, (New York: Democracy at Work, 2019), 29–39.
4. James Brown, "The Payback," *The Payback*, Polydor Records, 1973, accessed October 2025, Spotify.
5. Erich Fromm, *The Sane Society*, (London: Routledge & Kegan Paul Ltd, 1956), 30.
6. James Barnes, "The Politics of Distress: A Discussion with Dr. James Davies on His New Book 'Sedated,'" *Mad in the UK*, accessed October 2025,

https://www.madintheuk.com/2021/06/the-politics-of-distress-a-discussion-with-dr-james-davies-on-his-new-book-sedated/.

7. Gabriel Lopez-Garrido, "Bandura's Self-Efficacy Theory of Motivation in Psychology," *Simply Psychology*, May 1, 2025, accessed September 2025, https://www.simplypsychology.org/self-efficacy.html.

8. David J. Bergner, "Retired Priest and Clinician: President Trump Suffers from Narcissistic Personality Disorder," *Florida Today*, April 16, 2025, accessed September 2025, https://www.floridatoday.com/story/opinion/2025/04/16/opinion-trump-suffers-from-narcissistic-personality-disorder/83083830007/.

9. BBC, "How Many US Mass Shootings Have There Been in 2024?" *BBC News*, accessed September 2025, https://www.bbc.com/news/world-us-canada-41488081.

10. Mark Scolforo and Mike Catalini, "Adult Son Convicted, Sentenced to Life for Shooting and Beheading Father in Pennsylvania," *Associated Press*, accessed September 2025, https://apnews.com/article/father-beheaded-online-video-head-pennsylvania-mohn-ee1069e457493b47ea7601724a14a1a6.

11. R. Ghosh, "Danielle Johnson: LA Mom Who Stabbed Partner, Threw Daughters Out of the Car in Murder-Suicide Was Astrology Influencer and Feared World Would End with Eclipse," *International Business*

Times Singapore, accessed October 2025, https://www.ibtimes.sg/danielle-johnson-la-mom-who-stabbed-partner-threw-daughters-out-car-murder-suicide-was-74217.

Chapter 1

12. Kelly-Ann Allen, DeLeon L. Gray, Roy F. Baumeister, and Mark R. Leary, "The Need to Belong: A Deep Dive into the Origins, Implications, and Future of a Foundational Construct," *Educational Psychology Review* 34 (2022): 1138.
13. Allen et al., "The Need to Belong," *Educational Psychology Review*, 1137.
14. Rosemary K.M. Sword and Phillip Zimbardo, "Inside the Mind of White Supremacy," *Psychology Today*, September 6, 2020, accessed October 2025, https://www.psychologytoday.com/us/blog/the-time-cure/202009/inside-the-mind-of-white-supremacy.
15. Maria Trent, Danielle G. Dooley, and Jacqueline Douge, "The Impact of Racism on Child and Adolescent Health," *Pediatrics* 144, no. 2 (2019), American Academy of Pediatrics Policy Statement, accessed October 2025, http://publications.aap.org/pediatrics/article-pdf/144/2/e20191765/1077476/peds_20191765.pdf.
16. Trent, Dooley, and Douge, "The Impact of Racism on Child and Adolescent Health," *Pediatrics*, 2.

17. Megan Ravi, Sean Minton, and Sanne van Rooij, "Trauma and Its Widespread Impact on Black Communities," *Psychology Today*, August 31, 2022, accessed September 2025, https://www.psychologytoday.com/us/blog/outside-the-box/202208/trauma-and-its-widespread-impact-black-communities.

Chapter 2

18. Kaiser Family Foundation, "KFF/CNN Mental Health in America Survey," *KFF*, October 5, 2022, accessed September 2025, https://www.kff.org/mental-health/kff-cnn-mental-health-in-america-survey/.
19. Graham Peebles, "Mental Health Illness: A Global Tragedy by Design," *CounterPunch*, February 10, 2023, accessed September 2025, https://www.counterpunch.org/2023/02/10/mental-health-illness-a-global-tragedy-by-design/.
20. Benedict Carey, "Defying Prevention Efforts, Suicide Rates Are Climbing Across the Nation," *New York Times*, June 8, 2018, sec. A, p. 17.
21. Surgeon General of the United States, *Mental Health: A Report of the Surgeon General* (Washington, DC: U.S. Government Printing Office, 1999), ISBN 0-16-050300-0.
22. Eric Levenson, "Luigi Mangione's Supporters Say the Death Penalty 'Should Scare Anyone,'" *CNN*,

April 26, 2025, accessed September 2025, https://www.cnn.com/2025/04/26/us/luigi-mangione-supporters/.
23. Munira Z. Gunja, Evan D. Gumas, and Reginald D. Williams II, "U.S. Health Care from a Global Perspective, 2022: Accelerating Spending, Worsening Outcomes," *Commonwealth Fund*, accessed September 2025, https://www.commonwealthfund.org/publications/issue-briefs/2023/jan/us-health-care-global-perspective-2022/.
24. Joe Cronin, "The Best Health Care in the World: Country Rankings," *International Insurance*, accessed September 2025, https://www.internationalinsurance.com/health/systems/.
25. Brian Handwerk, "An Evolutionary Timeline of Homo Sapiens," *Smithsonian Magazine*, accessed September 2025, https://www.smithsonianmag.com/science-nature/essential-timeline-understanding-evolution-homo-sapiens-180976807/.
26. Rachelle Bradley, "An Introduction to the History and Principles of Traditional Homeopathic Medicine," *Heartland Naturopathic*, accessed September 2025, https://heartlandnaturopathic.com/an-introduction-to-the-history-and-principles-of-traditional-homeopathic-medicine/.
27. Claire Johnson and Bart Green, "100 Years After the Flexner Report: Reflections on Its Influence on Chiropractic Education," *Journal of Chiropractic Education* 24, no. 2 (2010): 146.

28. Eric Schmidt, "How Rockefeller Created the Business of Western Medicine," *Meridian Health Clinic*, accessed September 2025, https://meridianhealthclinic.com/how-rockefeller-created-the-business-of-western-medicine/.
29. David Edward Marcinko, "A Brief History of Managed Medical Care in the USA," *Medical Executive Post*, accessed September 2025, https://medicalexecutivepost.com/2024/05/06/a-brief-history-of-managed-care/.
30. "Transcript of Taped Conversation Between President Richard Nixon and John D. Ehrlichman (1971) That Led to the HMO Act of 1973," *Wikisource*, accessed September 2025, https://en.wikisource.org/wiki/Transcript_of_taped_conversation_between_President_Richard_Nixon_and_John_D_Ehrlichman_(1971)_
31. NAMI, "Mental Health Parity: Where We Stand," *National Alliance on Mental Illness*, accessed September 2025, https://www.nami.org/Advocacy/Policy-Priorities/Improving-Health/Mental-Health-Parity/.
32. Diana Novak Jones, "Trump Administration May Rescind Mental Health Parity Rule, Filing Says," *Reuters*, May 12, 2025, accessed September 2025, https://www.reuters.com/legal/government/trump-administration-may-rescind-mental-health-parity-rule-filing-says-2025-05-12/.

33. Deeya Prakash, "The Suicide Crisis Among Medical Providers—and How Health Care Leaders Are Combatting It," *Brown Public Health Journal*, accessed September 2025, https://sites.brown.edu/publichealthjournal/2024/03/21/the-suicide-crisis-among-medical-providers-and-how-healthcare-leaders-are
34. Wendy Dean and Matthew Ramsey, "How Insurers Hijacked the Doctor-Patient Relationship," *Health Care Uncovered*, accessed September 2025, https://healthcareuncovered.substack.com/p/how-insurers-hijacked-the-doctor.
35. Jeff Lagasse, "Class Action Lawsuit Against UnitedHealth's AI Claim Denials Advances," *Healthcare Finance News*, accessed September 2025, https://www.healthcarefinancenews.com/news/class-action-lawsuit-against-unitedhealths-ai-claim-denials-advances.
36. Andy Corbley, "Big Insurance Uses AI to Quickly Deny Claims, One Man Fights Back with AI App That Quickly Appeals," *Good News Network*, accessed September 2025, https://www.goodnewsnetwork.org/big-insurance-uses-ai-to-quickly-deny-claims-physican-fights-back-with-ai-app-that-quickly-appeals/.
37. Doug Smith, "The Toll of One Man's Mental Illness: 17 Criminal Cases, Six Competency Hearings, One Failed Conservatorship," *Los Angeles Times*, November 28, 2021, accessed September 2025,

https://www.latimes.com/homeless-housing/story/2021-11-28/column-one-toll-of-one-mans-mental-illness.
38. Samantha Schmidt, "A Violent, Mentally Ill Man Begged in Vain for Medication, Lawsuit Says. Then Three People Were Killed," *Washington Post*, November 17, 2017, accessed September 2025, https://www.washingtonpost.com/news/morning-mix/wp/2017/11/17/a-violent-mentally-ill-man-begged-in-vain-for-medication-lawsuit-says-then-he-
39. Mark Gokavi, "Dayton Triple Homicide Suspect Pleads Guilty, Avoids Death Penalty," *Dayton Daily News*, accessed September 2025, https://www.daytondailynews.com/news/crime--law/dayton-triple-homicide-suspect-plead-guilty-avoid-death-penalty/2cOS2vAFFqOvGphDSS9OtL/.
40. William Wan, "Is This What a Good Mother Looks Like?" *Washington Post*, March 17, 2022, accessed September 2025, https://www.washingtonpost.com/dc-md-va/2022/03/17/parental-rights-mental-illness-custody/
41. E. Fuller Torrey, "Ronald Reagan's Shameful Legacy: Violence, the Homeless, Mental Illness," *Salon*, September 29, 2013, accessed September 2025, https://www.salon.com/2013/09/29/ronald_reagans_shameful_legacy_violence_the_homeless_mental_illness/.
42. Bruce E. Levine, "Why Failed Psychiatry Lives On," *CounterPunch*, October 27, 2023, accessed Septem-

ber 2025, https://www.counterpunch.org/2023/10/27/why-failed-psychiatry-lives-on/print/.

43. Bruce E. Levine, "Scientific Misconduct and Fraud: The Final Nail in Psychiatry's Antidepressant Coffin," *CounterPunch*, January 17, 2024, accessed September 2025, https://www.counterpunch.org/2024/01/17/scientific-misconduct-and-fraud-the-final-nail-in-psychiatrys-antidepressant-coffin/print/.
44. Bruce E. Levine, "The Zyprexa Papers: A Legal System for Drug Companies and Lawyers... Not the Public," *CounterPunch*, September 4, 2020, accessed September 2025, https://www.counterpunch.org/2020/09/04/the-zyprexa-papers-a-legal-system-for-drug-companies-and-lawyers-not-the-public/print/.
45. Levine, "Why Failed Psychiatry Lives On," *CounterPunch*.
46. Robert Frank, "Meet the Private Doctor to the Wealthy—at $40,000 a Year," *CNBC*, April 22, 2024, accessed September 2025, https://www.cnbc.com/2024/04/22/meet-the-private-doctor-to-the-wealthy-at-40000-a-year.html.
47. Privé-Swiss, "Psychological and Emotional Treatment Program," *Privé-Swiss*, accessed September 2025, https://priveswiss.com/our-programs/psychological-and-emotional-treatment-program/.
48. Kaleigh Rogers, "I Went to a Therapist for the Wealthy to Find Out How Rich People Deal," *Vice*,

accessed September 2025, https://www.vice.com/en/article/i-went-to-a-therapist-for.

Chapter 3

49. Arthur S. Reber and Emily Reber, *The Penguin Dictionary of Psychology*, 3rd ed. (New York: Penguin Books, 2001), 157.
50. Maria Godoy, "You Can't Outrun a Bad Diet. Food – Not Lack of Exercise – Fuels Obesity, Study Finds," *NPR*, accessed September 2025, https://www.npr.org/2025/07/24/nx-s1-5477662/diet-exercise-obesity-nutrition.
51. Hoke S. Glover and V. Efua Prince, *Crazy as Hell* (New York: W.W. Norton, 2023), 19.
52. Glover and Prince, *Crazy as Hell*, 36.
53. Donovan Webster, "The Making of a Sniper," *Vanity Fair*, accessed September 2025, https://www.vanityfair.com/news/2004/10/beltway-snipers-200410.
54. Christopher Dorner, "To: America," accessed September 2025, https://laist.com/news/christopher-dorners-manifesto-in-fu.
55. Emma G. Gallegos, "Ex-LAPD Cop on Dorner's Manifesto: 'Not Only Do I Believe It, But I Lived It,'" *LAist*, accessed September 2025, https://laist.com/news/police-public-safety/another-ex-lapd-cop-speaks-out-agai.
56. Ian Ayres and Jonathan Borowsky, "A Study of Racially Disparate Outcomes in the Los Angeles Po-

lice Department," *ACLU of Southern California*, accessed September 2025, https://www.aclusocal.org/en/racial-profiling-lapd-study-racially-disparate-outcomes-los-angeles-police-department.
57. Aldo Salerno, "The Dark Side of American History, Part 5: Police Brutality in Los Angeles, 1950s to 1990s," *Substack*, accessed September 2025, https://asalerno.substack.com/p/the-dark-side-of-american-history-714.
58. Jessica P. Ogilvie, "Christopher Dorner's Manifesto in Full," *LAist*, Editor's Note dated June 12, 2020, accessed September 2025, https://laist.com/news/christopher-dorners-manifesto-in-fu.
59. Glover and Prince, *Crazy as Hell*, 19.
60. Adnan Hmidan, "Resistance Is Not a Democratic Option," *Palinfo*, accessed September 2025, https://english.palinfo.com/opinion_articles/resistance-is-not-a-democratic-option/.
61. Okan Keles, "The Poetic Way of Resistance to Western Hegemony: Where Fanon's Anti-Imperialism and Ismet Ozel's Spiritual Resistance Meet," *APA Blog*, accessed September 2025, https://blog.apaonline.org/2025/06/17/the-poetic-way-of-resistance-to-western-hegemony-where-fanons-anti-imperialism-and
62. Hamza Hamouchene, "Fanon and the Psychology of Oppression and Liberation," *CADTM*, accessed September 2025, https://www.cadtm.org/Fanon-and-the-Psychology-of-Oppression-and-Liberation.

63. Glover and Prince, *Crazy as Hell*, 58.
64. Juan Cole, "NOLA Attacker Was a Vet Who Fought the War on Terror Against Extremists Before Breakdown," *Informed Comment*, accessed September 2025, https://www.juancole.com/2025/01/attacker-extremists-breakdown.html.
65. Ty Roush, "Man Who Died in Cybertruck Explosion Identified as Green Beret and Bronze Star Recipient – Here's What We Know About Him," *Forbes*, accessed September 2025, https://www.forbes.com/sites/tylerroush/2025/01/08/man-who-died-in-cybertruck-explosion-identified-as-green-beret-and-bronze-star-recipient-heres-what-we-know-about-him
66. Kristie Rieken, "An Army Veteran's Path to Radicalization Followed Divorces and Struggling Businesses in Texas," *Associated Press*, accessed September 2025, https://apnews.com/article/new-orleans-terror-attack-driver-family-divorce-45a58097acfd821d44535fb5447f140d.
67. Chandelis Duster and Emma Bowman, "FBI Says the Suspect in the Deadly New Orleans Truck Attack Acted Alone," *NPR*, accessed September 2025, https://www.npr.org/2025/01/02/nx-s1-5245814/new-orleans-truck-attack-latest-fbi.
68. Seth Harp, *The Fort Bragg Cartel*, (New York: Viking, 2025), Kindle edition.
69. James C. Oleson, "A Requiem for the Unabomber," *Contemporary Justice Review* 26, no. 2 (2023): 171–199, accessed September 2025,

https://www.tandfonline.com/doi/full/10.1080/10282580.2023.2279312.
70. Bruce E. Levine, "The Tragedies of Ted Kaczynski," *CounterPunch*, accessed September 2025, https://www.counterpunch.org/2023/06/13/the-tragedies-of-ted-kaczynski/print/.
71. Erik Ortiz and Michael Kosnar, "'Unabomber' Ted Kaczynski Had Late-Stage Rectal Cancer and Was 'Depressed' Before Prison Suicide, Autopsy Says," *NBC News*, accessed September 2025, https://www.nbcnews.com/news/us-news/un-abomber-ted-kaczynski-late-stage-rectal-cancer-was-depressed-prison-rcna147819.

Chapter 4

72. Wade W. Nobles, *African Psychology: Toward Its Reclamation, Reascension & Revitalization* (Oakland: Black Family Institute, 1986), 94.
73. Nobles, *African Psychology*, 97.
74. Ipek S. Burnett, *A Jungian Inquiry Into the American Psyche: The Violence of Innocence* (New York: Routledge, 2020), 6.
75. Alexus McLeod, "Chinese Philosophy Has Long Known That Mental Health Is Communal," *Psyche*, accessed September 2025, https://psyche.co/ideas/chinese-philosophy-has-long-known-that-mental-health-is-communal.

76. Matt Huston, "The Upside of Dark Minds," *Psychology Today*, May/June 2013, 59.
77. M.E. Thomas, "Confessions of a Sociopath," *Psychology Today*, May/June 2013, 57.
78. Lisa Fritscher, "What Collective Unconscious Theory Tells Us About the Mind," *Verywell Mind*, accessed September 2025, https://www.verywellmind.com/what-is-the-collective-unconscious-2671571.
79. Joy DeGruy, *Post Traumatic Slave Syndrome: America's Legacy of Enduring Injury and Healing* (Portland: Joy DeGruy Publications, 2005), 264.
80. Neurolaunch Editorial Team, "Marxist Psychology: Exploring the Intersection of Socialism and Mental Health," *Neurolaunch*, accessed September 2025, https://neurolaunch.com/marxist-psychology/.
81. Joy DeGruy, "Post Traumatic Slave Syndrome," *Joy DeGruy Publications*, accessed September 2025, https://www.joydegruy.com/post-traumatic-slave-syndrome.
82. Vivek H. Murthy, "Our Epidemic of Loneliness and Isolation," *Office of the U.S. Surgeon General*, 2023, 4.
83. Elizabeth M. Ross, "What Is Causing Our Epidemic of Loneliness and How Can We Fix It?" *Usable Knowledge*, Harvard Graduate School of Education, accessed September 2025, https://www.gse.harvard.edu/ideas/usable-knowledge/24/10/what-causing-our-epidemic-loneliness-and-how-can-we-fix-

84. Murthy, "Our Epidemic of Loneliness and Isolation," 16.
85. Murthy, "Our Epidemic of Loneliness and Isolation," 16.
86. Murthy, "Our Epidemic of Loneliness and Isolation," 51.
87. Daniel Kruger, "Social Media Copies Gambling Methods 'to Create Psychological Craving,'" *University of Michigan Institute for Healthcare Policy & Innovation*, accessed September 2025, https://ihpi.umich.edu/news/social-media-copies-gambling-methods-create-psychological-cravings.
88. Mike Allen, "Sean Parker Unloads on Facebook: 'God Only Knows What It's Doing to Our Children's Brains,'" *Axios*, accessed September 2025, https://www.axios.com/2017/12/15/sean-parker-unloads-on-facebook-god-only-knows-what-its-doing-to-our-childrens-brains-1513306792.
89. Jon Johnson and Amy Murnan, "8 Negative Effects of Technology," *Medical News Today*, accessed September 2025, https://www.medicalnewstoday.com/articles/negative-effects-of-technology.
90. Gary Goldfield, "The Effects of Social Media Use on Teen's Body Image," *Psychology Today*, accessed September 2025, https://www.psychologytoday.com/us/blog/no-more-fomo/202312/the-effects-of-social-media-use-on-teens-body-image.
91. Meharry School of Global Health, "The Projected Costs and Economic Impact of Mental Health In-

equities in the United States," accessed September 2025, https://www.meharryglobal.org/wp-content/uploads/2024/05/DI_CHS_Cost-of-MH-inequities.pdf.
92. Quan Nguyen, "Why We Should Nationalize Social Media," *Caraid*, accessed September 2025, https://caraid.stir.ac.uk/2017/12/08/why-we-should-nationalise-social-media/.

Chapter 5

93. Tulane University Celia Scott Weatherhead School of Public Health, "Understanding Mental Health as a Public Health Issue," accessed September 2025, https://publichealth.tulane.edu/blog/mental-health-public-health/.
94. Tulane University, "Understanding Mental Health as a Public Health Issue."
95. Anna Gorman, "Use of Psychiatric Drugs Soars in California Jails," *California Healthline*, accessed September 2025, https://californiahealthline.org/news/number-of-california-jail-inmates-on-psychiatric-drugs-soars/.
96. Gorman, "Use of Psychiatric Drugs Soars in California Jails."
97. Patrick Cockburn, "Treating Mental Health Patients as Criminals," *CounterPunch*, accessed September 2025, https://www.counterpunch.org/2017/04/24/

treating-mental-health-patients-as-criminals/print/.

98. Marlena Batchelor, "The Best Countries for Mental Wellbeing," *The CEO Magazine*, accessed September 2025, https://www.theceomagazine.com/business/health-wellbeing/countries-with-the-best-mental-health-care/.

99. National Center for Injury Prevention and Control, "Protecting the Nation's Mental Health," *CDC*, accessed September 2025, https://www.cdc.gov/mental-health/about/what-cdc-is-doing.html.

100. Gene Ira Katz, "Rethinking Law Enforcement Approaches to Mental Health Crises," *APB Web*, accessed September 2025, https://apbweb.com/2024/10/rethinking-law-enforcement-approaches-to-mental-health-crises/.

101. Johns Hopkins Bloomberg School of Public Health, "Study of Fatal and Nonfatal Shootings by Police Reveals Racial Disparities, Dispatch Risks," accessed September 2025, https://publichealth.jhu.edu/2024/study-of-fatal-and-nonfatal-shootings-by-police-reveals-racial-disparities-dispatch-risks.

102. Lynne Peeples, "What the Data Say About Police Shootings," *Scientific American*, accessed September 2025, https://www.scientificamerican.com/article/what-the-data-say-about-police-shootings/.

103. Brita Belli, "Racial Disparity in Police Shootings Unchanged Over 5 Years," *Yale News*, accessed September 2025, https://news.yale.edu/2020/10/27/

racial-disparity-police-shootings-unchanged-over-5-years.
104. Julianne McShane, "Report: Police Killings Rose in the Five Years After George Floyd's Murder," *Mother Jones*, accessed September 2025, https://www.motherjones.com/politics/2025/05/george-floyd-police-killings-blm/.
105. NAMI, "Crisis Intervention Team (CIT) Programs," *National Alliance on Mental Illness*, accessed September 2025, https://www.nami.org/Advocacy/Crisis-Intervention/crisis-intervention-team-cit-programs/.
106. Michael S. Rogers, Dale E. McNiel, and Renee L. Binder, "Effectiveness of Police Crisis Intervention Training Programs," *Journal of the American Academy of Psychiatry and the Law* 47, no. 4 (2019), accessed September 2025, https://doi.org/10.29158/JAAPL.003863-19.
107. Katrina Pross, "More Cities Remove Police from Teams Responding to Mental Health Crisis Calls," *Side Effects Public Media*, accessed September 2025, https://www.sideeffectspublicmedia.org/mental-health/2023-10-30/more-cities-remove-police-from-teams-responding-to-mental-health-crisis-calls.
108. Rogers, McNiel, and Binder, "Effectiveness of Police Crisis Intervention Training Programs."
109. Pete Earley, "LA NAMI Chapter Questions Death by Police: Warn of Cutbacks to CIT Training," accessed September 2025, https://www.peteearley.com/

2020/10/05/la-nami-chapter-questions-death-by-police-warn-of-cutbacks-to-cit-training/.
110. Lauren Victoria Burke, "Mayor Scott Condemns Trump Administration's Cuts to Public Safety Funding," *Black Press USA*, accessed September 2025, https://blackpressusa.com/mayor-scott-condemns-trump-administrations-cuts-to-public-safety-funding/.
111. Philip Lukens, "How President Trump's Recent Actions Could Impact Law Enforcement," *Police1*, accessed September 2025, https://www.police1.com/chiefs-sheriffs/how-president-trumps-recent-actions-could-impact-law-enforcement/.
112. Ashleigh Hollowell, "Proposed Trump Budget Reveals $28.6B in Cuts to Behavioral Health Science Related Agencies," *Behavioral Health Business*, accessed September 2025, https://bhbusiness.com/2025/05/05/proposed-trump-budget-reveals-28-6b-in-cuts-to-behavioral-health-science-related-agencies/.
113. William Cooper, "Which Countries Are the Best for Mental Health," *William Russell*, accessed September 2025, https://www.william-russell.com/blog/countries-best-mental-healthcare/#countries.
114. Kate E. Pickett and Richard G. Wilkinson, "Inequality: An Underacknowledged Source of Mental Illness and Distress," *The British Journal of Psychiatry* 197 (2010): 426–428, https://doi.org/10.1192/bjp.bp.109.072066.

115. Manuel E. Yepe, "How Capitalism Erodes Mental Health," *CounterPunch*, accessed September 2025, https://www.counterpunch.org/2018/08/21/how-capitalism-erodes-mental-health/print/.
116. Stephen Prager, "'The System Is Rigged': CEOs Made 285 Times More Than Their Workers in 2024: AFL-CIO Report," *Common Dreams*, accessed September 2025, https://www.commondreams.org/news/afl-cio-ceo-pay-report.
117. Khanyi Mlaba, "The Richest 1% Own Almost Half the World's Wealth & 9 Other Mind-Blowing Facts on Wealth Inequality," *Global Citizen*, accessed September 2025, https://www.globalcitizen.org/en/content/wealth-inequality-oxfam-billionaires-elon-musk/.
118. Lauren C. Davis, Alexa T. Diianni, Sydney R. Drumheller, Noha N Elansary, Gianna N. D'Ambrozio, Farahdeba Herrawi, Brian J. Piper, Lisa Cosgrove, "Undisclosed Financial Conflicts of Interest in DSM-5: Cross Sectional Analysis," *British Medical Journal* 384 (2024): e076902, , accessed September 2025, https://doi.org/10.1136/bmj-2023-076902.
119. Christopher Lane, "The NIMH Withdraws Support for DSM-5," *Psychology Today*, accessed September 2025, https://www.psychologytoday.com/us/blog/side-effects/201305/the-nimh-withdraws-support-for-dsm-5.
120. Blake Griffin Edwards, "System for Mental Health Diagnosis Is Corrupt, Some Experts Say," *Psychology*

Today, accessed September 2025, https://www.psychologytoday.com/us/blog/progress-notes/202001/system-mental-health-diagnosis-is-corrupt-some-experts-say.

Chapter 6

121. F. Douglas Stephenson, "Beware of Health Insurance Companies Bearing Gifts," *CounterPunch*, accessed September 2025, https://www.counterpunch.org/2025/08/20/beware-of-health-insurance-companies-bearing-gifts/print/.
122. Jessica Corbett, "'Gouging': US Health Insurance Giants Raked in Over $71 Billion in Profits Last Year," *Common Dreams*, accessed September 2025, https://www.commondreams.org/news/health-insurance-profits.
123. Mindhelp, "Do You Have Good Mental Health?" accessed September 2025, https://mind.help/topic/what-is-good-mental-health/.
124. Julia Neuberger, "Let's Do Away with 'Patients,'" *National Center for Biotechnology Information*, accessed September 2025, https://pmc.ncbi.nlm.nih.gov/articles/PMC1116090/.
125. Merriam-Webster Dictionary, "The History of 'Doctor,'" accessed September 2025, https://www.merriam-webster.com/wordplay/the-history-of-doctor.

126. Megan Brenan, "Majority in U.S. Still Say Gov't Should Ensure Health Care," *Gallup*, accessed September 2025, https://news.gallup.com/poll/468401/majority-say-gov-ensure-health-care.aspx?version=print.
127. Scott Tucker and Larry Gross, "The Sabotage of Single Payer Health Care," *CounterPunch*, accessed September 2025, https://www.counterpunch.org/2025/09/07/the-sabotage-of-single-payer-health-care/.
128. Martin Gillens and Benjamin Page, "Testing Theories of American Politics: Elites, Interest Groups, and Average Citizens," accessed September 2025, https://archive.org/details/gilens_and_page_2014_-testing_theories_of_american_politics.doc.
129. Tucker and Gross, "The Sabotage of Single Payer Health Care," 37–38.

Chapter 7

130. Sarah Peters Kernan, "Sugar and Power in the Early Modern World," *Newberry Digital Collections*, accessed September 2025, https://dcc.newberry.org/?p=16944.
131. Gabriella Gershenson, "A Brief and Bizarre History of Artificial Sweeteners," *Saveur*, accessed September 2025, https://www.saveur.com/artificial-sweeteners/.

132. Leo DeLuca, "Before Folding 30 Years Ago, the Sears Catalog Sold Some Surprising Products," *Smithsonian Magazine*, accessed September 2025, https://www.smithsonianmag.com/innovation/before-folding-30-years-ago-the-sears-catalog-sold-some-surprising-products-180981504/.
133. Joseph Detrano, "The Four Sentence Letter Behind the Rise of Oxycontin," *Rutgers Center of Alcohol Studies*, accessed September 2025, https://alcoholstudies.rutgers.edu/the-four-sentence-letter-behind-the-rise-of-oxycontin/.
134. Centers for Disease Control and Prevention, "Understanding the Opioid Overdose Epidemic," accessed September 2025, https://www.cdc.gov/overdose-prevention/about/understanding-the-opioid-overdose-epidemic.html.
135. Fran Quigley, "How Corporations Killed Medicine," *CounterPunch*, accessed September 2025, https://www.counterpunch.org/2016/02/09/how-corporations-killed-medicine/.
136. Niall McCarthy, "Which Companies Received the Most Covid-19 Vaccine R&D Funding?" *Forbes*, accessed September 2025, https://www.forbes.com/sites/niallmccarthy/2021/05/06/which-companies-received-the-most-covid-19-vaccine-rd-funding-infographic/.
137. Catherine Madden, Benjamin Black, and Debra Willsie, "Treating Our Youngest Patients: Psychotropic Medications in Early Childhood," *Na-

tional Center for Biotechnology Information*, accessed September 2025, https://pmc.ncbi.nlm.nih.gov/articles/PMC6179566/.

138. Ronan McGreevy, "An Irish Doctor on Why She Believes Autism, ADHD and Depression Are Being Overdiagnosed," *Irish Times*, accessed September 2025, https://www.irishtimes.com/health/your-family/2025/04/05/adhd-children-are-now-in-a-queue-with-50-year-old-adults-for-a-drug-that-is-in-s

139. Christopher Lane, "ADHD Is Now Widely Overdiagnosed and for Multiple Reasons," *Psychology Today*, accessed September 2025, https://www.psychologytoday.com/us/blog/side-effects/201710/adhd-is-now-widely-overdiagnosed-and-multiple-reasons.

140. IQVIA Government Solutions, "Stimulant Prescription Trends in the United States 2012–2023," accessed September 2025, https://deadiversion.usdoj.gov/pubs/docs/IQVIA-Report-on-Stimulant-Trends-2024.pdf.

141. Philip Hickey, "The Drugging of Children in Foster Care," *Mad in America*, accessed September 2025, https://www.madinamerica.com/2015/03/drugging-children-foster-care/.

142. Robert T. Muller, "Antidepressants and Teen Suicide," *Psychology Today*, accessed September 2025, https://www.psychologytoday.com/ca/blog/talking-about-trauma/201305/antidepressants-and-teen-suicide.

143. Bonnie Burstow, "Psychiatric Drugging of Children and Youth as a Form of Child Abuse: Not a Radical Proposition," *Springer Publishing*, accessed September 2025, https://connect.springerpub.com/highwire_display/entity_view/node/79816/full.
144. Juan Cole, "Psychopathocracy 3.0," *Informed Comment*, accessed September 2025, https://www.juancole.com/2025/08/psychopathocracy-3-0.html.
145. Steve Taylor, "In the Seat of Pathocracy," *Psychology Today*, November/December 2019, 30.
146. Oliver James, "Selfish Capitalism Is Bad for Our Mental Health," *SOTT.net*, accessed September 2025, https://www.sott.net/article/146622-Selfish-capitalism-is-bad-for-our-mental-health.
147. Eric W. Dolan, "Emotional Distress Among Voters Tied to Trump's Populist Appeal, Research Shows," *PsyPost*, accessed September 2025, https://www.psypost.org/emotional-distress-among-voters-tied-to-trumps-populist-appeal-research-shows/.
148. Thomas F. Pettigrew, "Social Psychological Perspectives on Trump Supporters," *Journal of Social and Political Psychology* 5, no. 1 (2017): 107–116, https://doi.org/10.5964/jspp.v5i1.750.
149. Editors, "New Poll: Democratic Socialism Is Now Mainstream," *Jacobin*, accessed September 2025, https://jacobin.com/2025/09/new-poll-democratic-socialism-mainstream.

Chapter 8

150. Manrado Gorgio, "Rollerball Is Still a Chillingly Relevant Science Fiction Movie Worth Your Time," *Science Fiction Classics*, accessed September 2025, https://www.sciencefictionclassics.com/rollerball-is-still-a-chillingly-relevant-science-fiction-movie-worth-your-time/.
151. Jessica Koehler, "Wired for Positivity: How Optimism Shapes Our Well-Being," *Psychology Today*, accessed September 2025, https://www.psychologytoday.com/us/blog/beyond-school-walls/202409/wired-for-positivity-how-optimism-shapes-our-well-being.
152. Wolff, *Understanding Socialism*, 122–123.
153. Wolff, *Understanding Socialism*, 120.
154. Brands Owned By, "Who Owns Publix: Top Shareholders," accessed September 2025, https://brandsownedby.com/who-owns-publix/.
155. Tod Perry, "If the Total Amount of Money Held by Americans Was Distributed Evenly, How Much Would You Get?" *Upworthy*, accessed September 2025, https://www.upworthy.com/economic-equality-ex.
156. The Neuron, "The Rise of the Robots: How Automation Is Changing the World," *Quantum Zeitgeist*, accessed September 2025, https://quantumzeitgeist.com/the-rise-of-the-ro-

bots-how-automation-is-changing-the-world/#10-job-displacement-and-economic-impact.
157. Alberto Garzon, "The Paradox of Progress: Why Do We Work So Much in the Age of Technology?" *Substack*, accessed September 2025, https://agarzon.substack.com/p/the-paradox-of-progress-why-do-we.
158. Richard D. Wolff, "AI: Profit vs. Freedom," *CounterPunch*, accessed September 2025, https://www.counterpunch.org/2023/09/25/ai-profit-vs-freedom/print/.
159. David Kabali Masembe, "Key Assumptions of Microeconomics Explained," *KnowledgePlusDK*, accessed September 2025, https://knowledgeplusdk.wordpress.com/2025/01/03/key-assumptions-microeconomics-explained/#Perfect.
160. Scott Nevil, "Understanding Fractional Reserve Banking: How It Fuels Economic Growth," *Investopedia*, accessed September 2025, https://www.investopedia.com/terms/f/fractionalreservebanking.asp.
161. Jill Schulman, "Embrace the Suck, Bravery's a Skill. Here's How to Do Hard Things," *Psychology Today*, September/October 2025, 44.

Chapter 9

162. David Hackworth, "David H. Hackworth Quotes," *Goodreads*, accessed September 2025,

https://www.goodreads.com/author/quotes/96212.David_H_Hackworth.
163. Edward Tick, *War and the Soul* (Wheaton, IL: Quest Books, 2005), 155.
164. Tick, *War and the Soul*, 108.
165. Tick, *War and the Soul*, 210.
166. C.L.R. James, *The Black Jacobins* (New York: Vintage Books, 1963), 418.
167. Frantz Fanon, *The Wretched of the Earth* (New York: Grove Press, 1966), 238.
168. Fanon, *The Wretched of the Earth*, 254.
169. Aaron T. Beck, *Prisoners of Hate* (New York: Harper Collins, 1999), 248.
170. Beck, *Prisoners of Hate*, 245.
171. Gwendolyn Brooks, "Paul Robeson," *Poets.org*, accessed October 2025, https://poets.org/poem/paul-robeson/print.
172. Leen Aghabi, Neven Bondokji, Aletha Osborne, and Kim Wilkinson, "Social Identity and Radicalization: A Review of Key Concepts," *WANA Institute*, accessed October 2025, https://wanainstitute.org/sites/default/files/publications/Publication_SocialIdentityTheory_English.pdf.
173. Middle East Eye Staff, "US TikTok Ban Linked to Pro-Palestine Content Rather Than China Threat, Insiders Reveal," *Middle East Eye*, accessed October 2025, https://www.middleeasteye.net/news/us-tiktok-ban-linked-israel-china-insiders-reveal.

174. Nardos Haile, "As the Clock Ticks for TikTok, Users Can Migrate to Numerous Alternatives," *Salon*, accessed October 2025, https://www.salon.com/2025/01/16/as-the-clock-ticks-for-tiktok-users-can-migrate-to-numerous-alternatives/.
175. Carlos L. Garrido and Edward Liger Smith, "Pioneers for Communism: Strive to Be Like Che," *Popular Resistance*, accessed October 2025, https://popularresistance.org/pioneers-for-communism-strive-to-be-like-che/.
176. Ernesto Guevara, "On Revolutionary Medicine," *Marxists Internet Archive*, accessed October 2025, https://www.marxists.org/archive/guevara/1960/08/19.htm.

Chapter 10

177. Karl Marx, *Economic and Philosophic Manuscripts of 1844* (New York: International Publishers, 1964), 112–113.
178. Centers for Disease Control and Prevention, "Health Effects of Social Isolation and Loneliness," accessed October 2025, https://www.cdc.gov/social-connectedness/risk-factors/index.html.
179. Carlos Todd, "The Difference Between Anger and Resentment," *Mastering Anger*, accessed October 2025, https://masteringanger.com/blog/difference-between-anger-and-resentment/.

180. Tricia Hersey, *We Will Rest! The Art of Escape* (New York: Little, Brown Spark, 2024), 84–85.
181. Hersey, *We Will Rest!*, 103.
182. bell hooks, *All About Love* (New York: William Morrow, 2001), 197.

www.ingramcontent.com/pod-product-compliance
Lightning Source LLC
Chambersburg PA
CBHW020459030426
42337CB00011B/155